PEERLESS

How to Slow Your Aging,
Grow Younger,
& Live Well Into the 22nd Century

Marc D. Baldwin, PhD

Peerless

© 2021 Marc D. Baldwin, PhD

Paperback ISBN: 978-1-66780-334-0

eBook ISBN: 978-1-66780-335-7

Dedication

Thanks family—without you, nothing means anything.

TABLE OF CONTENTS

FOREWORD

"How old would you be if you didn't know how old you was?"

—*Satchel Paige (1906-1982)*

"The wiser mind mourns less for what age takes away

than what it leaves behind."

—*William Wordsworth (1770-1850)*

Day 1: July 21, 2020

I woke up this day at 4:42 AM. Couldn't sleep anymore. I lay in bed next to my beautiful wife, feeling blessed but profoundly different because this was my 70th birthday.

Some birds chirped, our cat meowed out on the patio, my wife stirred, yet the pre-dawn darkness prevailed. All so normal.

But me?

I took a long deep breath and asked myself the cliched rhetorical question: How did I get this old? And the only answer I could come up with is this: I survived.

Then it hit me like the proverbial ton of bricks: **I want to survive for a whole lot longer. I don't want to be 70 years old. I don't want to be an "old man." I don't want to die. I want to live another 70 years or more.**

I swung my body around out of bed, put my feet on the floor, stood up, stretched out my arthritic back, and just stood there, by my bed, by my sleeping wife, while the birds chirped and the cat meowed, and all was normal.

But I was now 70 years old. 70.

I did the only thing I can do about it: I got some cold water and cold coffee and went back to work on this book I started just the day before. Literally, on July 20th, I got inspired and got to work writing this book.

We Can Live Well Into the 22nd Century

Thanks to some good books I'd been reading, I became convinced on 7/20/20 that rather than getting weaker and older, I could, in fact, get stronger *and younger*. Of course, I'd already known that stronger could be done, but younger? That's a pipe dream, right? Wrong.

I spent all day on the 20th doing more research into it—reading dozens of websites, articles, and many more book summaries and reviews (of books I've since bought and read) on Amazon. The more I read, the more I became convinced that we *actually can* make our minds and bodies younger, at least biologically, if not in actual age.

Not only can old age be treated and postponed in many ways, but it can also be reversed.

Whether we're 20 or 90 years old, the *PEERLESS* system I detail in this book may well help us live until we're 125 or even older. And not just live, but live well, live productively —live as much younger people than our actual ages would suggest.

My goal is to live to 150. I'm taking all bets.

I'm starting now by writing this book. The hardest part of anything is starting.

The encouraging news is that we're not starting too late or alone. We're starting in the nick of time. And we've got a lot of help, guidance, and inspiration from many brilliant scientists and doctors who've been at this anti- and reverse aging quest for 25 years or more.

Meet the Anti-Aging Dream Team

Dr. Michael Fossel, Dr. Aubrey de Grey, Dr. Judith Campisi, Dave Asprey, and Dr. David Sinclair—just to name a few—are some of the world's cutting-edge longevity experts, Daniel Boones scouting the new frontier and blazing the trail toward extending the human lifespan.

Fossel's landmark book, *Reversing Human Aging* (1996), was the first of its kind ever written about how aging works and how to reverse it.

de Grey and his co-author Michael Rae followed up with *Ending Aging* (2008), positing that the key biomedical technology to *"end death entirely... is now within reach."*

Since the early 1990s, Campisi, a professor at the world-famous Buck Institute and founder of *Unity Biotechnology*, has been working on "taming cellular senescence," the source of chronic inflammation implicated in all major diseases.

Asprey—the world's #1 biohacker—states that his goal is to live to at least 180. After reading his book *Super Human: The Bulletproof Plan to Age Backward and Maybe Even Live Forever* (2019), I'm convinced that the concept of aging backward is absolutely rational and scientifically proven.

The thesis of Sinclair's book, *Lifespan: Why We Age—and Why We Don't Have To* (2017), is this astounding statement:

> I believe that **aging is a disease**. I believe it is treatable. I believe we can treat it within our lifetimes. And in so doing, I believe, everything we know about human health will be fundamentally changed. (p. 81)

That's excellent news for everybody, especially Seniors in declining health.

"Making 90 the New 50 By 2030" is the tagline of de Grey's Methuselah Foundation (www.mfoundation.org). His institute is just one of several institutes working on reverse aging. Comprised of doctors, scientists, and investors, they *"incubate and sponsor mission-relevant ventures, fund research, and support projects and prizes to accelerate breakthroughs in longevity."* The plan is that by the time today's 40-year olds reach 80 in 2060, it's possible they'll feel like 40 for a long time—perhaps living until they're 200 or older.

In Chapter 8, Singularity and Science, I'll be detailing what these scientists and others are doing to make that dream of a longer life a reality within the next 10-15 years. Medical science—with an assist from Artificial Intelligence (AI)—is fast identifying the root causes of aging and developing reverse aging magic medicines, treatments such as cellular reprogramming, and miraculous nanorobots to circulate through our bloodstreams (to name just a few breathtaking advances).

The Bottom Line?

If you're 30 years old now, you might live another 150 years. Although Seniors like me might not have another 150 years in us, we might have 50 or 75 more years. At the very least, we can definitely break the 125-year-old barrier, the glass ceiling of humanity's longevity.

How Exactly *Can* We Live Well Into the 22ⁿᵈ Century?

By whipping ourselves into peak mental and physical shape right now. Only top gun, right stuff kind of people become astronauts and get to ride rocket ships to the moon.

This *PEERLESS* system is that moon-shot vehicle, the top gun training, the right stuff system to take us to the 22nd century and beyond.

I've crafted this system from hundreds, if not thousands of books, theories, methods, breakthroughs, breathtaking insights, and practical strategies. Distilling those lessons down into this Reader's Digest, condensed version of how we can take charge of our lives and maximize our health and lifespan.

This is not pie-in-the-sky speculation, pseudo-science, or con-man quackery. This is real, valid, proven science.

The thesis of the scientific research and work behind reverse aging, and this book about it, is so revolutionary, it bears repeating: **Within the next 10-15 years, the scientific breakthroughs *will be*—not *may be*, but *will be*—so mind-boggling, even 85 or 90-year-olds will be reversing their aging and living healthy, strong, and productive lives well into their hundreds.**

> *I have little doubt that cellular reprogramming is the next frontier in aging research.... If we can fix the toughest to fix and regenerate the toughest to regenerate cells in our body, there's really no reason to suspect we cannot regrow any type of cells our bodies need. Yes, that could be fixing fresh spinal cord injuries, but it also means regrowing any other kind of tissue in the body that has been damaged by age: from the liver to the kidney, from the heart to the brain. Nothing is off the table.* (Sinclair, p. 172)

It Sounds Too Good to Be True…So What's the Catch?

The catch, for Seniors at least, is that we'll have to be reasonably healthy and fit 85 or 90-year-olds to avail ourselves of such miracle cures. *"Doubling the human lifespan—which is entirely feasible—can only be done by ensuring that we live in good health,"* notes Dr. Fossel (p. 190).

If we're barely hanging on, reverse aging probably won't work for us. But if we start growing mentally and physically stronger and younger *right now,* we can be lively and looking great when the Times Square ball drops on 2100.

In fact, in his conclusion, Dr. Fossel doubles down: *"We can at least double the human lifespan and will likely extend the average lifespan to several centuries of active, healthy life"* (p. 191). We can live for *"several centuries"*?! Wow!

Get ready to party on New Year's Eve 2099!

Methodology & Structure

Before we begin, a few quick details about my methodology and the book's structure are in order:

Why *PEERLESS*? It's an acronym: **P**roduce, achieve **E**quanimity, **E**at right, **R**ead, **L**earn, **E**xercise, **S**ustain, and make it to the (double **S**) **Singularity** when medical **Science** can reverse our aging and help us live well into the 22nd Century.

The Acronym as Mantra

Many authorities on self-development and high performance suggest creating an acronym or mantra to repeat to ourselves to keep us on track and focused. So I came up with PEERLESS because that seems like a good way to be.

I've arranged the letters to spell out the word "peerless," obviously, yet perhaps you might find that it would be better for you to start with the letter **E**. Maybe everything begins with managing your emotions, achieving equanimity, and envisioning success. Or start with **S** for Science because that's the chapter about your health conditions and the scientific/medical research about how to prevent, properly treat, and even reverse aging through this entire process, as well as many recommended supplements to complement your diet. Or start with **L** because learning is a fundamental key to making it all work out right. It really doesn't matter much what order you go over the elements. But the acronym *PEERLESS* is an easy, quick mantra for me to mentally run through all the ingredients to keep myself on track and focused.

Housekeeping

Here are some other random details about how I keep this book neat and orderly.

<u>Caps and whatnot</u>

I often capitalize and italicize or bold words throughout the book <u>that would not ordinarily be capitalized or italicized.</u> I do so to call our attention to them as concepts to focus on and read more about in our research. For example, *Equanimity* and *Mindfulness* are two ideas that, if you're anything like me, have rarely crossed your mind throughout your life. But once you embrace them, they're fascinating and fruitful states of mind to pursue 24/7.

<u>Emojis and Symbols</u>

Since we can remember and internalize concepts, ideas, and systems much more effectively with acronyms, <u>lettered shorthand, and symbols</u>, I'll pose

Questions ?, and provide Takeaways ☞, Actions 𝄫, Obstacles ⊘ to beware of along your way, and recommendations of books you Must Read 📚.

No Blank Pages or Exercises and Such

Unlike many other books such as mine, <u>I don't provide blank pages for you nor demand you do something immediately.</u> I'll expect you to do what you want when you want. You decide how much or how little you'll embrace this system. For example, when I ask questions, I'll give you my answers and hope you'll then provide your own answers. I can't force anyone to be peerless. Until early in 2020, I couldn't even force myself.

Fortunately for me, something clicked on 2/4/2020 when I started to lose weight and then clicked into high gear on 7/20/2020 when I *really* started getting focused. I'll talk about that later. But, the takeaway is this: You've got to provide your own "click," answer your own questions, review and even research the takeaways, use the Tools, and then plan and manage your answers and actions.

INTRODUCTION

The System is the Solution

— AT&T

I'm convinced that the best and perhaps the only way we can succeed is to stick to a system. Personally, I need a practical, daily routine to stay on track. It wakes me up in the morning and keeps me going all day. Without it, I'm prone to drift and meander.

So, here's my *PEERLESS* system. It's working for me, and I know it'll work for you too.

> **P = Produce**. We need to stay busy producing, immersing ourselves in Projects. We can't waste any time, stagnate, or let a single day go by without working on producing a better self for ourselves. Creating gives us a Purpose. It's our One Big Thing. We need to make Progress every day. As I'm polishing this section on 8/3/20, I realize I've been writing this book for only 2 weeks now. In just 2 weeks, I've got 35 pages. It's rough, and I've a long way to go with both this first draft and all subsequent drafts. But I'm making Progress.

E = Equanimity. Be balanced, steady, and calm. Nurture Mindfulness through conscious breathing, Meditation, and paying attention to what we're paying attention to.

E = Eat right. Lose weight. Get on a low carb (only good carbs) and zero (or close to zero) sugars diet. Get as healthy as humanly possible.

R = Read. Put down our phones. Turn off the TV. Read. It's calming, motivational, inspirational. Read insightful books to support and enhance this Plan. Reading recharges us.

L = Learn. Exercise our brains. Never stop growing mentally and spiritually; strive to be wise. Learning wards off aging.

E = Exercise. Get to the gym 5-6 days a week. Run. Jog. Power walk. Bike ride. Swim. Stretch. Stand. Move. Get in the best shape of our lives.

S = Sustain. Keep it going every minute of every day. Don't lose momentum by having bad days. Having a bad day is not an option. Convert bad days into good days through mental strength and fortitude. Sustaining this system is essential to its ultimate success.

S = Singularity and Science. Medical science—particularly the science of longevity and reverse aging—is now so advanced. It's fascinating and imperative to learn how we actually *can* live well into the 22nd century if only we try.

So…Happy 70th Birthday to Me!

PEERLESS is my birthday gift to myself: my determination to become peerless. My 70th birthday is a reset, a new beginning, a rebirth, Year One.

I invite you to put aside your skepticism and doubts, and join me on our quest toward growing younger.

CHAPTER 1

Produce

Produce! Produce!

— Ralph Waldo Emerson

The essence and foundation, the alpha and omega of being *PEERLESS*, is to stay busy, producing all that you possibly can. Civilization began with the production of fire, shelter, tools, and then agriculture, progressing into laws, human rights, and democracy. They were all productions.

Everything that defines us as different from lower animals is a production. This entire system—every system—is a production.

You are a production. Staying busy every day, eating right, exercising, prioritizing, and planning for a healthier, stronger you in the near future by sustaining your efforts to learn about and utilize medical Science—it's all a production.

We have the power to produce whatever life we want for ourselves. Whatever *self* we envision for ourselves, we can produce that *self.*

The goal of this entire system is to live a better, healthier, longer life. And **it starts with recognizing that we need to produce that result for ourselves.**

As Dr. William Davis argues in his seminal work *Undoctored*, we *cannot* rely on the medical community to make us healthier or help us live longer lives. That's *not* their main goal.

> *… By taking the reins of health care of yourself, you are not trying to avoid a gleaming, efficient, and charitable system set up to serve you. You are trying to avoid being exploited, abused, and misled by a system driven by perverse motivations, unjustifiable costs, and incomplete protections, shaking you down for money like a mafia leg-breaker at every opportunity while claiming to follow a calling or be your guardian angel making you believe you will be sunk without them.* (Davis, p. 43)

That may sound like a grossly unfair characterization of the healthcare industry, but it's the grim reality that Davis convincingly details. Big Pharma, hospitals, and doctors—whether nefariously or inadvertently—have produced for themselves a vast money-making machine totally reliant upon people becoming and remaining sick. Their conglomerated production sucks us in and keeps us there. <u>Consequently, it's up to each of us to produce our own good health, our own long lives.</u>

Please understand that I'm *not* saying that *your* doctors are bad people who don't care about you. They're likely very good people who *do* care about you. But the system itself has serious issues. Good people can be compromised by bad systems.

It's become popular in the 2020s to talk about "systemic" problems with this or that issue. That's what's happened to the healthcare system: it's a huge, complex, messy, flawed system that often—not always, but often—makes it very difficult for good doctors to do a good job.

That's why we need to help our doctors out by taking charge of our own health through understanding, monitoring, and controlling what we eat, how we stay in shape, why our bodies are afflicted with our own personal health problems, and what we can do to address them and prevent further problems from developing.

In Chapter 8, I'll return to a thorough discussion of all the marvels Science has produced and will soon produce to help us become healthier and live longer.

But first, let's start by building our foundation: the production values, plans, priorities, principles, and mindset that will prepare us to utilize that Science.

How Did I Produce *PEERLESS?*

After reading many books and brainstorming hundreds of important necessities and ingredients to having a successful, long life, I arrived at a lot of questions that I've attempted to answer:

?

- How long do you want to live?
- How healthy do you think you need to be to live that long life?
- What else do you want for your long life than just a long life?
- How would you define your life right now?
- To date, what has been your life's work?
- What would you like your life's work to be?
- What should be your legacy?

As I've said, my answers to the first two questions are these: I want to live to 150, and I can't do that unless I'm very healthy *and* productive, since good health *requires* us to be productive—a symbiotic relationship I'll discuss in this chapter.

My answers to the next five questions comprise the essence of this chapter.

Necessity is the Mother of Invention—We *Need* to Be Productive

We all want to leave behind when we're gone things both tangible and intangible: good memories of us in our loved ones' minds and hearts, as well as tangible things, such as property, wealth, or a company, a business, etc. Some of us would like to leave behind books or songs we've written, a house we've built or crafted, various objects of arts and crafts we've enjoyed and mastered, perhaps furniture or a car or a cabin we've built. Actual physical projects we've seen to fruition with our own brain and hands. Products of our labor. Productions we've envisioned and made real.

As human beings, we *need* to produce, be productive, make our lives a production. We *need* to produce ourselves, lest others dictate and determine our lives for us.

We could all benefit from being more like Walt Whitman's *"Noiseless, patient spider"*:

A noiseless patient spider,

I mark'd where on a little promontory it stood isolated,

Mark'd how to explore the vacant vast surrounding,

It launch'd forth filament, filament, filament, out of itself,

Ever unreeling them, ever tirelessly speeding them.

And you O my soul where you stand,

Surrounded, detached, in measureless oceans of space,

Ceaselessly musing, venturing, throwing, seeking the spheres to connect them,

Till the bridge you will need be form'd, till the ductile anchor hold,

Till the gossamer thread you fling catch somewhere, O my soul.

<u>We have everything we need inside us</u> to create, connect, and catch hold of life before it's gone. We just need to work at it. Work on us. Work the system, and it will work for us.

When we get rolling with the work, it becomes a pleasure.

> *My object in living is to unite*
> *My avocation and my vocation*
> *As my two eyes make one in sight.*
> *Only where love and need are one,*
> *And the work is play for mortal stakes,*
> *Is the deed ever really done*
> *For Heaven and the future's sakes*
>
> (from "*Two Tramps In Mud Time*" by Robert Frost)

Producing, having projects, staying busy is good for our brains, our cognitive health. Ray Kurzweil, the author of *The Singularity is Near*, warns that "*by failing to engage it in intellectually challenging activities, your brain will fail to grow new connections and it will indeed become disorganized and ultimately dysfunctional*" (*Transcend*, p. 8).

Personally, I need both a good, strong body and brain to attain my ultimate goal, which is to reach my 80s and then 90s as a healthy, fit, productive man, both for myself and for my family. I don't want to be an aged, decrepit, sickly burden on my family.

I'm determined to be a longevity pioneer, one of the first to live to 125 and beyond—to at least 150. Does that sound delusional, crazy, impossible? Sure. I know it does. But, it can happen. In fact, people *will be* living to 150 and older. I'm aiming to be one of them.

So, in a very real sense, the main production of every day forward—for me and for you too, I hope—is ourselves. We must do us. Not only for us, but for our families. And even society. The world needs good people to live longer.

On a plane, if the air masks deploy in an emergency, the first thing everyone must do is secure the air mask on their own faces. Then, after *you* are breathing the air, you can help others around you who may need assistance in securing their air masks. Only when *you* are secure can you effectively help others be secure.

For *my* security, being productive will lead to living longer. Staying busy and producing results is the driving force, the first and most essential fundamental in achieving success in every letter of the PEERLESS system. We simply must produce results or we fail. No production = no success.

But exactly how do we stay busy producing? How do we get more things done than ever before? By following a system, a routine, a schedule. By managing our actions.

> *The key to managing all of your stuff is managing your actions....The substantive issue is how to make appropriate choices about what to do at any point in time. The real work is to manage our actions....the real problem is a lack of clarity and definition about what a project really is, and what associated next-action steps are required.* (Allen, pp. 20-21)

Managing our actions throughout the rest of this chapter:

1. Start by Writing

    1. Mission Statement

    2. Goals

    3. Action Plans

4. Journal

5. Strengths and Skills inventory

6. Must Improve list

2. Get to work

🖉 **Write. That's right: we should write. I'll even go further: we *must* write.**

Develop the Habit of Writing

This entire *PEERLESS* system may be challenging to embrace and follow, but I bet the writing part might be the hardest for many of us. If we're not active writers, we have to learn to be. Writing is essential to our success.

You don't have to write an article, a blog, or a book about what you know as well or better than anyone else. But it would benefit you tremendously to do so.

Seriously. Writing is a production that benefits you in more ways than I can count. I could write an entire book about why you should write a book.

Here are just a few benefits of writing: it's cathartic, therapeutic, mentally stimulating, creative, meaningful, and fun. It organizes and structures you. It keeps you accountable to you.

My #1 frustration in life now is not having enough time to produce, to write this book, specifically. I'm getting upset by how much else I have to do during the day that keeps me from producing this book. Of course, almost everything else I do during the day is related to this *PEERLESS* system, so I don't waste too much time. My priorities are centered around my family, as always: but for myself, writing this book reinforces me. It organizes me. It structures me. It keeps me on track and focused.

Still not sold on the idea of writing? Well, start selling yourself on the idea. While you're working your way up to writing a book, start with smaller projects.

This new chapter in your *PEERLESS* life should include a goal of writing every day. You are choosing the words to describe exactly who you are, both to yourself and to the world, for the present and the future.

> *Words are powerful. They set expectations and limits and send messages to our brains and even our bodies about how much we are capable of. Language is a part of your mental software. Use it consciously and with precision, and you will achieve things you probably never thought you could. (Asprey, Game Changers, p. 19)*

Write These Now!

Whether or not you ever write an article, blog, or book, <u>I urge you to write the following</u> 6 texts ASAP:

1. Your Mission Statement (MS

2. Your Goals (G)

3. Your Action Plans (A)

4. Your Journal (J)

5. Your Skills and Strengths Inventory (SSI)

6. Your Must Improve List (MIL)

Note that I say *your* MS, G, A, J, SSI, and MIL. They are *your* personal writing projects, which form the fundamental record of everything you need to concretize in writing. You're contracting with yourself when you write these texts. Get it down in writing, and you exponentially improve your chances of succeeding.

Mission Statement: Your Personal Declaration and Constitution

Essential to our focus is to craft our own personal MS. It is our condensed and concise manifesto for living. Why are we alive? What is our life's mission? In his masterpiece, *The 7 Habits of Highly Effective People*, Stephen Covey notes that

> *A personal mission statement or philosophy or creed focuses on what you want to be (character) and to do (contributions and achievements) and on the values or principles upon which being and doing are based.... It becomes a personal constitution, the basis for making major, life-directing decisions, the basis for making daily decisions in the midst of circumstances and emotions that affect our lives.* (Covey, p. 106 & 108)

I thought long and hard about it. More than anything, I want to continue to have a profound and positive effect on my family.

What you leave behind is not what is engraved in stone monuments, but what is woven into the lives of others.—Pericles

My Personal MS

With that goal being my primary focus, here's my personal MS:

To better care for, nurture, and defend my wife, kids, grandkids, and myself, I will spend the rest of my life trying to become PEERLESS.

- *I will follow my PEERLESS system every day.*

- *I will make myself as physically and mentally strong as possible.*

- *I will be a model of a principled man, fostering and ever-increasing my integrity, honesty, self-discipline, fortitude, compassion, equanimity, love, and sacred honor.*

- *I will plan tomorrow's work today.*

- *I will not waver from this MS.*

Goals

Over the past 15-20 years, I've read more than 200 self-help, personal development, motivational books. (Apparently, I've always needed a lot of help and motivation…lol). Every single one of those books had a section, chapter, or at least a passing reference to the importance of making goals and writing them down.

Goal setting is beginning with the end in mind, which is *"based on the principle that* all things are created twice. *There's a mental or first creation, and a physical or second creation to all things"* (Covey, p. 99).

When she was 12 years old, one of my amazing daughters announced that she'd made up her mind about what she was going to do with her life. "I've decided my goal is to get my college degree in computer graphics and then move to Hollywood to work in the movies right after graduation." "Great, darling," I said, smiling and hugging her. A proud father of his darling and delightful daughter. It's not that I took her announcement lightly or doubted her, but she was 12. She'd always been as precocious as can be. How could she really expect such a goal to be realized just as she'd planned it in 6th grade? Well, 10 years later, my family and I were in the audience cheering her as she walked across the stage and accepted her college degree in computer graphics. Three days after that, we loaded a rental truck with all of her stuff and drove her across the country to her new apartment in Hollywood. That Monday, she started her new job working in the movies. My wonderful daughter made her dreams come true by deciding on her goals at the age of 12 and working from then on to make them a reality.

My step-daughter and son-in-law also knew what they wanted—each other. They met in high school, fell in love, and were inseparable. At the ages of 16 and 17, they decided then to get college degrees, good jobs, get married, and have kids. They achieved all those goals and now have a house in one of Florida's best beach towns. AND, best of all, they have three truly wonderful little boys—our grandchildren. I'm so proud of them and those terrific kids. Everything they wanted they got by working hard and staying the course.

While I'm at it, I'd be remiss, not to mention my stepson. He also knew what he wanted and is well on his way to getting it—a career as a movie maker/screenwriter/director. From the time he was 7, he was making Halloween haunted houses in his room. By 12, he was writing and making movies. Now at 22, he's on a scholarship in film school on his way to—I'm sure—making it in Hollywood. All because he had a dream, a plan, a goal for himself that he worked on every day.

When you set goals for yourself, you're **making decisions** about what sort of *self* you are creating to be *your* self.

Tony Robbins writes inspirationally about the "consciousness-awakening" power of making decisions:

> Making a true decision means committing to achieving a result, and then cutting yourself off from any other possibility.... ***It's your decisions about what to focus on, what things mean to you, and what you're going to do about them that will determine your ultimate destiny.*** (Robbins, pp. 39-40)

<u>Goal setting is all about making decisions.</u> Once you make those decisions, you significantly increase your chances of achieving your goals if you concretely and expressly set them in stone by writing them down.

In fact, our brains have a mechanism known as the Reticular Activating System (RAS) that *"determines what you will notice and what you will pay attention to. It is the screening device of your mind....Once you decide that something is a priority, you give it tremendous emotional intensity, and by continually focusing on it, any resource that supports its attainment will eventually become clear"* (Robbins, pp. 287-88).

Operating like a computer, our brains process what's entered into them. They even have a self-activating search function that monitors our behavior. Once we program our brains with written MS, Goals, and Action Plans, we can count on our RAS to keep us focused.

> *Your automatic creative mechanism is teleological. That is, it operates in terms of goals and end results. Once you give it a definite goal to achieve, you can depend upon its automatic guidance system to take you to that goal much better than "you" ever could by conscious thought. "You" supply the goal by thinking in terms of end results. Your automatic mechanism then supplies the means whereby. (Maltz)*

A common-sense strategy recommended by everyone from Mark Twain to Navy SEALS is to <u>reduce complex tasks into smaller, more manageable tasks</u>. Do the first one and then the second and so on. Don't be overwhelmed by the size and scope of any project. Simply cut it down to bite-sized pieces and get to work.

> *If you try to solve every problem or complete every task simultaneously, you will fail at all of them. Pick the biggest problem or the issue that will provide the most positive impact. Then focus your resources on that and attack*

it. Get it taken care of. Once you have done that, you can move on to the next problem or issue, then the one after that. Continue doing that until you have stabilized the situation. Prioritize and execute. (Willink, from Ferriss, *Tribe of Mentors*, p. 539)

To start, I made a list of my long-term goals. I used 5 years as a long-term. Then, I broke them down into 1 year, 1 month, 1 week, and daily goals. Then, I wrote specific, actionable plans. I revised the following Goals on 8/6/20:

<u>5-year goals:</u>

- To have stuck to everything in my *PEERLESS* system.
- To have tripled my income (from my online business)
- To have written 5 books
- To have a muscular physique

<u>1-year goal:</u>

- To have finished PEERLESS and begun a 2nd book
- To have increased my business income by 50%
- To have reached an optimum weight of 195 or less.
- To have increased my gym time to 1.5 hours 4-5x per week.
- To have made progress in reducing my body fat and attaining a 6-pack.

<u>1-month goal:</u>

- To have stuck to PEERLESS every day
- To have finished 50% of this book
- To have lost 5 more pounds, down to 205 or less.

<u>1-week goal:</u>

- To have stuck to PEERLESS all week

- To have lost 1-2 pounds

- To have written every day

Once we write down our goals, we need to devise our plan of action. As the inimitable Seth Godin sagely notes: *"...action is easy once you have a plan. Formulating a plan, however, is a rare and valuable skill"* (*Poke the Box*, p. 63).

Tony Robbins encouragingly adds that *"Giant goals produce giant motivation....All goal setting must be immediately followed by both the development of a plan, and massive incessant action toward its fulfillment"* (Robbins, p. 272 & 275).

<u>My Action Plans:</u>

- Get plenty of sleep

- Wake up and get to work by 6 AM at the latest

- Drink lots of water, do stretches, think through the day

- Morning meditation

- Get to work

- Get my business emails done first

- Then work on this book for as long as possible, a minimum of 2 hours.

- Then the gym

- Throughout the rest of the day:

    o Review PEERLESS, my mantras, MS, and daily, weekly, monthly goals.

    o Full-scale meditation

o Stay attentive to the course. Don't lose focus. Write more, read more, record my thoughts and progress in my journal.

o Review and work on other tasks and projects, all related to PEERLESS.

o Give my entire family love and attention.

🎬 Time to get to work! Write your MS, Goals, & Action Plans. It was my experience that once I formulated my MS and set my Goals and Action plans, I was highly motivated to get going. I hope you feel the same way!

Constantly Monitor & Revise Your Goals If Need Be

Once we've written down our MS, Goals, and Action Plans, our *"RAS will become sensitized as you consistently review your goals and reasons, and will attract to you any resource of value to the achievement of your clearly defined desire"* (Robbins, p. 302).

While I was in the gym this morning (8:00-9:00 am, 8/5/20), I was working my plan, being mindful, meditating my mantras and *PEERLESS*, and going over my goals; I couldn't shake the feeling of being troubled about something. I've been struggling with a problem, and I couldn't bring myself to identify it. But it finally hit me: I need to pay more attention to addressing my son's attention, MS, goals, moods, attitude, etc. He's a great kid, but he wastes too much time and doesn't like to read. Too much iPhone and not enough production.

So I resolved then and there to take charge and teach him about being *PEERLESS*. To do so, I first needed to revise my weekly and monthly goals, and even my MS, to include him. To prioritize him and his mental education.

He will be starting 10th grade in 12 days. So my goal is to get him on a schedule.

I don't want to be looking back at these months we had together, beating myself up about having failed to improve his habits and skills. I have 12 days. 12 days to get him on a schedule of reading and being productive, writing an MS and goals, writing in his journal daily.

I, the teacher, must teach him about being *PEERLESS*.

So, here are my revised **Goals** for this week and next week:

- Continue with my own *PEERLESS* system, sharing it with my son
- Maintain all my current goals, sharing them with my son
- Teach my son to write an MS
- Teach my son to write down his Goals
- Teach my son to write in his journal every day
- Read a variety of motivational articles and passages from some of the books I'm reading

(9/23/20 Update: We did it all. We achieved everything on the Goals list and had fun doing it!)

Habits: Break Bad Habits, Make Good Habits

Winners master fundamentals. In Fall football training camps and baseball Spring Training, the very best professional players, the men who've been playing football and baseball since they were 4 years old, return to practicing the fundamentals with endless blocking, tackling, pass routes, fielding, throwing, and hitting drills. Back to basics. They want to win.

Everyone wants to win. Everyone *needs* to win. That's what we're doing here: trying to win. *Planning* to win.

The only way we can all win—the only way anyone can become peerless—is to master their particular system's fundamentals. And fundamentals are habits. The right habits. **Habits are fundamental to winning, fundamental to success in life.**

Success, however you define it, is achievable if you collect the right field-tested beliefs and habits. (Ferriss, Tools, p. XXII)

On the football and baseball fields, the players' beliefs and habits are tested and perfected. In our lives, we're developing the habits of staying busy, producing, following an MS, pursuing Goals, creating Action Plans to keep us on track, and writing it all down. These habitual behaviors exponentially increase our chances of winning.

We first make our habits, and then our habits make us.—John Dryden

Covey defines a habit *"as the intersection of knowledge, skill, and desire. Knowledge is the theoretical paradigm, the what to do and the why. Skill is the how to do. And desire is the motivation, the* want *to do. In order to make something a habit in our lives, we have to have all three"* (p. 47).

In this book and system, I'll provide a lot of knowledge and explain how to attain many of the necessary skills. I'll also pump us up with motivational talk and techniques. But it's all ineffective if we don't apply the knowledge, learn the skills, and stay motivated without constant babysitting. **Like everything else, it's all up to us. We have to buy-in.**

World-famous high-performance coach Brendon Burchard also extols the importance of developing the right habits: *"High performance is not achieved by a specific kind of person, but rather by a specific set of practices, which I call high performance habits"* (Burchard, p. 12).

During his career of training people how to be "extraordinary," Burchard conducted extensive research—really impressive studies, surveys, before-and-after programs, assessments, reviews, and more—that concluded: *"High performers have simply mastered—either on purpose or by accident through necessity—six habits that matter most in reaching and sustaining long-term success. We call these six habits the HP6. They have to do with clarity, energy, necessity, productivity, influence, and courage"* (p. 21).

The important point here is that success depends upon practicing the right habits.

We are what we repeatedly do.

> *Excellence, then, is not an act, but a habit.*
> — Aristotle

Do the Work—Repeatedly

Now that our MS, Goals, and Action Plans are set, and we understand the necessity of making and maintaining the right habits, we need to be like Aristotle and repeatedly do our work. Get to it and we will be rewarded with inspiration.

> *When we sit down day after day and keep grinding, something mysterious starts to happen. The process is set in the motion by which, inevitably and infallibly, heaven comes to our aid. Unseen forces enlist in our cause; serendipity reinforces our purpose....When we sit down each day and do our work, power concentrates around us. The Muse takes note of our dedication. She approves. (Pressfield, p. 108)*

Stephen Pressfield is talking about art—writing or painting or some other artistic endeavor. However, it applies to any sort of work. Don't be put off if you don't believe in God, heaven, or the Muse. Just substitute the supernatural, the unknown, the inexplicable. Fate. Fortune. Whatever works for you. Just do the work every day. That's the message. It's so true, so real, often mysterious, but definitely in play. When you do your work, your work will do you.

Concentrate all your thoughts upon the work at hand.

The sun's rays do not burn until brought to a focus.

— Alexander Graham Bell

Daily Journal Writing

<u>What to Journal?</u> I use journaling to record everything: how my book is going, how I feel, what I've done and plan to do next, random observations and thoughts, lists of things to do, and general recording of my life.

<u>When to Journal?</u> Throughout the day. I start first thing in the morning, after drinking water, stretching, and meditating on my day: my Goals, my focus, my *PEERLESS* mantra, my MS. Then, after I've pre-written—gone through it in my mind—I journal, recording everything quickly and concisely into my Google Doc (Gdoc).

An Aside About Google Docs (Gdocs)

If you are not already using Google Docs—or similar software to create multiple documents for yourself—consider doing so. First, you need a Gmail email address. Then you'll have access to Google Drive and Google docs. Gdocs are robust tools to stay organized. I have one for everything: this book, notes on this book, a To-Do list, my Bibliography, important information and records, comprehensive information on the editors who work with my company, and many more. You can keep them all available in tabs on your toolbar so that you can toggle easily and instantly back and forth to any one of them you need at that moment. AND you can access them all on your smartphone! You can copy and paste material, move it from one doc to another, even share any specific doc you want with anyone else who has them. For example, if you want to share your doc with your wife or colleague, you can each have access to it and use it simultaneously in real-time. They're an essential organizing system for my business and life. I highly recommend them.

<u>Where to journal?</u> I journal at my desk into my Gdoc. But I also journal into my Gdoc using my phone app and voice dictation anywhere and everywhere an idea comes to me.

When I say "journal," I also mean simply "write." In addition to working on my daily journal (or diary, if you will), I also work on my books—this one and future additional writing projects. I just "wrote" between several sets at the gym. I had some good ideas for material, so I dictated them into my *PEERLESS* Gdoc.

So, whether you're journaling or writing, the concept to embrace and develop into an ongoing, anytime, anywhere habit is just to write and <u>write as much and often as you can.</u>

<u>Why journal or write at all?</u>

I'm hoping this is self-evident to you, but if not, briefly: writing a journal and an article, blog, or book is producing yourself. Writing is developing you. Putting your thoughts in writing—whether in an MS, goal setting, journaling, or writing a book—clarifies you to yourself. It concretizes you. Reinforces you. In a very real sense, your writing writes you. You come into better focus and reality for yourself. Your writing creates you.

By writing down our thoughts and plans prior to starting the day's real work of turning the thinking, plans, goals into doing them, we get reinforced, focused, and determined.

Journaling is a kind of envisioning, a visualization of sorts. We see what we want to do then we write it down.

An extra bonus of writing is what surfaces that we hadn't even thought of consciously. The very process of writing is deep thinking. New ideas or clarifications and crystallizations pop up like magic. Writing is cathartic and exploratory. In writing, we become and create ourselves. It's a discourse with ourselves.

> *The bedrock tool of a creative recovery is something I call Morning Pages: three pages of longhand, morning writing about absolutely anything. They are to be written first thing in the morning, and shown to no one. There is no wrong way to do Morning Pages. I like to think of them as windshield wipers, swiping away anything that stands between you and a clear view of your day. (Cameron)*

How to write? Just do it. It doesn't have to be perfect. Consider everything you write a rough draft. You just need to put in the work. Get words down on paper (or, more efficiently, especially for rewriting, adding, crafting, polishing, editing) using a Gdoc. Larry Page, the co-founder of Google, said that partially succeeding has not been appreciated. You don't have to have a 100% smashing success. Just create a partial success and then keep working on it.

I hold a Ph.D. in English (more specifically, composition and literature), and I taught writing and literature for 40 years in high school and college. I always told my students to just get words on paper. Don't worry about grammar, punctuation, even the best diction or sentence structure. Just get it down. You can proof it and make it better later. Writing is rewriting.

You're spitballing, brainstorming, teaching yourself how to write. Most importantly, you're talking to yourself as you write. You're pumping yourself up and giving yourself a talking to. You're doing you.

A Skills/Strengths Inventory (S/SI)

What is a S/SI?

A list of your own skills, strengths, and productions in life so far.

?

- What have you made?

- What can you do?

- What are you good at?

- What do you like to do?

- What projects have you got going, or have you always wanted to get going?

- Are you good with tools?

    o A handyman?

    o A carpenter?

    o A mechanic?

Look around your house, your community, your kids' school, even where you work (or worked if you're retired). Can you volunteer? What needs to be done? What's in a state of disrepair? Why not take it upon yourself to help out or lead the way if no one else is?

Getting going on a project will stimulate your brain and body. Producing something will produce a better, stronger you. A project is a projection of you. You, in fact, *are* the project. As you work and produce, the project produces you.

There is a fountain of youth: it is your mind, your talents,

the creativity you bring to your life and the lives of people you love.

When you learn to tap this source, you will truly have defeated age.

— Sophia Loren

?

Have you always worked more with your head than your hands?

- Are you a banker, investor, teacher, doctor, lawyer, business owner, salesman?

- What are your fundamental skills and strengths?

What projects can you plan and get busy on that employ your greatest talents?

Why write a S/SI?

Because the #1 thing you need to understand is yourself. Who are you? *"Know thyself"* is the timeless advice inscribed in the temple of Delphi in Greece more than 2400 years ago. We don't really *know* too many people by what they say. We know them by what they *do* or can do: by their actions, their job, their family, their productions. Learn who you are—at least a good part of who you are—by inventorying your skills, your strengths.

My S/SI:

- A Ph.D. in English

- I can read, write, teach, and edit pretty well.

- I've written some published articles and books.

- I had a good teaching career; thousands of students told me I was good, and hundreds of written evaluations confirmed my quality.

- I founded an online editing service, doing all my own editing for the first year or so until I started hiring others to do it for me.

Those are my base income-earning skills. But what else can I do? What other strengths do I have?

- I can make a plan and stick to it.

- I get excited and pumped up when I'm staying busy.

- I love life and want to live to 150 or more.

- I'm compassionate, generous, energetic, giving, caring, decent, and devoted.

- I would die to protect my loved ones.

- I'm resilient, optimistic, and determined to make the most of every second of every day.

I have many (though not all) of the inherent attributes necessary to achieve my goals successfully. But what can I do to nurture and grow what I lack or need more of? *PEERLESS* can help me do that.

And lest you believe—based on the preceding S/SI—that I think too highly of myself, I really don't. I've got a long way to go. Keep reading, and you'll see that I know I'm a work-in-progress (WIP).

A Must Improve List (MIL)

What is a MIL? An honest, no-holds-barred self-assessment of what you lack to achieve your *PEERLESS* self.

Why write a MIL? For the same reasons that we're writing an SSI: we need to know who we truly are. No more dancing around the truth about what's wrong with us.

?

- What's wrong with you?

- What do people criticize about you? Not that everyone's right in their criticism, but if they have something negative to say about you, it's possible, isn't it, that they may be right?

- What's been holding you back?

- Why are you overweight, broke, having personal problems?

Be honest with yourself. Make this list from the perspective of your worst enemy. Face facts. We need to fix our flaws, or at least acknowledge and attempt to address them. Tough to do? Yes, very. So, I'll go first.

My MIL:

Up until July 20th, 2020, when I became inspired to write this book, I had deluded myself for 69 years and 364 days. I'd always thought I'd be healthy, wealthy, and wise by the time I hit 70. But I'm barely healthy, certainly not wealthy, and only on occasion, wise. I can be arrogant and often obnoxious. I sometimes talk too much and say things I regret. I complain and, too often, make excuses. I sometimes procrastinate, get lazy, or even get down. And sometimes, I lose my temper: an anger management problem. I did have a good career as a professor, so I thought that was it. I had settled for cruising along, doing what I could with my life that remains, just taking care of my family and my business. I'd resigned myself to my current situation of being less than I should be. I failed to see a way out and up—a path I could take to have a better life and become a better man. I'd given up and in.

As an aside I'll develop in Chapter 2, Eating, I actually began my transformation on February 4, 2020. On that date, I started my Weight Watchers diet, exercise routine, and journal. By July 20, 2020, I'd lost 35 pounds and was doing much better. But I still lacked focus, drive, determination. I was still wallowing in the willy-nilly land of not having distinct goals or knowing what I was going to do with the rest of my life.

But now, I've faced my flaws and created a Mission Statement, Goals, and Action Plans for myself. I'm developing new habits. I'm 100% committed to fixing—or at least addressing, reducing, and persistently attacking—my flaws. I *will* be a better person.

Okay. I just ripped myself to shreds, so now it's your turn. Rip yourself to shreds. Really let yourself have it. And after you've written that confession to yourself about yourself, resolve to make yourself a better person.

Brainstorm and make your own list of productions that will benefit your family, your friends, and your community—not just or solely yourself. Why? Because what we do for others makes us happier and more fulfilled than what we do solely for ourselves. Karma. What goes around, comes around. Pay it forward.

Here's a wildly ambitious project to consider: go way out of your comfort zone and consider doing a TED talk. TED Talks are presentations by experts (in education, business, science, tech, and the creative arts), given at TED conferences, filmed, and turned into free videos. See https://www.ted.com/talks.

The one and only Seth Godin poses the challenge:

- *If you had a chance to do a TED talk, what would it be about?*

- *What have you discovered, what do you know, what can you teach?*

- *You should do one. Even if you don't do one, you should be prepared to do one. That's your opportunity to approach your work in a way to generate unique learning and interactions that are worth sharing. (Poke the Box, p. 41)*

Hey, it's worth considering, even if you would never actually present it at a TED conference. Just *considering* doing a TED talk is an excellent way of focusing in on your #1 skill and area of expertise. Think hard on this question: Do you have a great story to tell about your particular set of skills? I bet you do. And even if you never do an actual TED talk, you can write your story and see where it takes you.

In fact, as I mentioned earlier, you *should* write a book. You've got one or more in you. Think about it.

Supplemental/Corollary Ps

The letter **P** just happens to be rich with other words relevant to the subjects we've just discussed. So let's add these words to our mantra: Purpose, Principles, Proactive, Plan, Prioritize, Process, Pleasure and Pain, Persist, and Progress.

When we run through *PEERLESS* in our mind for the first few weeks, we should add these other **P's** to Produce, thereby activating instant recall and giving us that much more to guide us. Is this strategy somewhat forced, artificial, or arbitrary? Sure. But it's a proven method to *mantracize* our thoughts and scan quickly through not just the 8 focal aspects of *PEERLESS*, but through several more within a minute or two.

☞ **I cannot overestimate the power of the mantra when repeated fast and focused several times a day**. As I said, after doing this for 2-3 weeks, the system and all its key points should be ingrained into us. After that, we probably won't need to continue the rote repetition—though I still run through the letters a lot myself, often while working out at the gym.

☞ The reason for this repetition of the key words and concepts is that **our minds will commit to what they pay attention to**. Paying immediate attention to your mantra's many focusing terms shapes them into unbreakable habits. (See my discussion of Paying Attention in Chapter 3, Equanimity).

<u>Know Your Purpose</u>

More studies than can be mentioned conclude that people who believe they have a Purpose in life live a better life—happier, more fulfilled, more "successful" in many measurable ways.

Your purpose should dictate what you spend your energy and time on. Doing things that you decide are important, such as those on your MS and Goals, will increase your happiness and satisfaction, and thus, have a ripple effect on everything else you do that day, that week, and throughout your entire life.

What is your Purpose? You should have expressly stated it in your MS. Sometimes called "Your One Big Thing," your Purpose guides and steadies you, focuses you. You can use it as a mantra and recall it anytime you need to get back on track.

The purpose of life is a life of purpose.

— Robert Byrne

My Purpose is this: To be a model father, husband, and grandfather, held up by my family as a rock and shining example of how to conduct yourself through life. A gentleman and a scholar. A kind, compassionate, yet strong Type A man who can be counted on in both daily moments and severe crises. The one to turn to. The gentle and tender nurturer and the savage warrior. Basically, the patriarch who will never let you down.

That's a lot to aspire to. I may well fall short in total and on many occasions. But that's my Purpose and my Goal for the rest of my life.

Live by Principles

The bedrock of our behavior should be principles. It seems self-evident to me. Without unchanging principles, we're at the mercy of every internal and external wind that blows us about. Our guiding principles should be integrity, honesty, self-discipline, fortitude, compassion, equanimity, love, and sacred honor. You can easily add many more to that list. They should be addressed in our MS. *"A personal mission statement based on correct principles...becomes a personal constitution, the basis for making major life-directing decisions..."* (Covey, p. 108).

Be Proactive

The essential thesis of *The 7 Habits* is that we should be proactive in how we face and address every situation, every interaction, everything that happens to us during the day. Do not *react* to what other people say or do or don't say or don't do. Seek mindfulness, equanimity: a calm, centered approach to every second of the day (See Chapter 3).

Being proactive *"means that as human beings, we are responsible for our own lives. Our behavior is a function of our decisions, not our conditions. We can subordinate feelings to values. We have the initiative and the responsibility to make things happen"* (Covey, p. 71).

The proactive mindset is similar to Jocko Willink's Navy SEAL stance of *Extreme Ownership: "Own it all,"* he says (from Ferriss, *Tools*, p. 415).

Jocko brings extreme ownership to everything, even or especially the worst life has to offer:

> *How do I deal with setbacks, failures, delays, defeat, or other disasters? I actually have a fairly simple way of dealing with these situations. There is one word to deal with all those situations, and that is: 'good.'...That's it. When things are going bad, don't get all bummed out, don't get startled, don't get frustrated. No. Just look at the issue and say: 'Good.'...accept reality, but focus on the solution. Take that issue, take that setback, take that problem, and turn it into something good. Go forward....If you can say the word 'good,' guess what? It means you're still alive. It means you're still breathing. And if you're still breathing, that means you've still got some fight left in you. So get up, dust off, reload, recalibrate, re-engage, and go out on the attack. And that, right there, is about as good as it gets. (from Ferriss, Tools, pp. 640-641)*

Good. That's the ticket. *It's all good.* Bring it on and handle it proactively.

Jocko Willink's *Extreme Ownership.* I believe that Jocko's quote is all the sales pitch the book needs.

Stephen Covey's *7 Habits of Highly Effective People* is one of the Top 5 best self-help, motivational books ever written. It's pure genius. Get it and read it. I could fill up this book with his quotes and methods, but then this book would just be a regurgitation of the *7 Habits.* It's that good.

<u>Always be Planning</u>

You must make plans, lists, get organized and structured constantly, add to them, tweak them, flesh them out. Putting it in writing is essential to getting it done.

<u>Prioritize Constantly</u>

As I just said, it is essential to prioritize your day and your week and your month. You need to get into the habit of putting first things first.

When Jocko Willink is feeling overwhelmed or unfocused, he

> *...prioritizes and executes. I learned this in combat. When things are going wrong, when multiple problems are occurring all at once, when things get overwhelming, you have to prioritize and execute. Look at the situation and assess the multitude of problems, tasks, or issues. Choose the one that is going to have the biggest impact and execute on that. (from Ferriss, Tribe, p. 539)*

Covey developed his Time Management Matrix, a 4-quadrant method of categorizing our daily activities based on urgency and importance. Urgent/Important activities must be handled first. Urgent/Not Important activities are often time wasters that get our attention nonetheless: interruptions, some calls, some emails, some other activities we like to do. Not-urgent/unimportant activities get far too much attention from us (trivia, busy work, other time-wasters).

The 2nd quadrant of Important/Not-urgent is where we procrastinate, yet self-development falls into this category. In fact, most of the *PEERLESS* activities could be categorized as important but not urgent. We need to revise our thinking and instill a sense of urgency in such matters as working on our goals, exercising, reading and learning, and making progress on this system. (See Covey, p. 146-182)

📖 Every day should begin by revisiting our goals and attending to the most important ones, even if they don't seem urgent. I've composed this mantra to help me pay attention to what's truly important: *"I will work on me with a sense of urgency. I cannot wait for me to get better and better."*

Trust the Process

The system is a process. Trust the process. You might not have your mind entirely made up yet. You might have those doubts and fears. But you just need to accept that it's a process. By working the process, your mind will come around.

Many people believe

> *that you first have to change your mind before you can change anything else. That you have to find balance before you can run....but this is exactly backward—that the surest way to change attitude is to change behavior....we derive our attitudes from how we behave, and figure out who we are by watching what we do. (Matthews, p. 72)*

Eugene "Mercury" Morris, the great running back of the undefeated 1972 Miami Dolphins, understands this principle well.

I lived in Ft. Lauderdale from 1963-1984. My buddies and I were there during the perfect season of 1972. We went to every game. It was glorious. 1973 was good too. But in 1974, we noticed that Merc was slower, not making the cuts around the ends as he'd done in previous years. Turns out, Merc had discovered cocaine.

When he first tried cocaine, his mind wasn't into it. But then, after he got hooked, his mind followed along. He was convicted in 1982 and served time for drug dealing, though he claimed he was set up. He didn't deny he was a user, but maintains even today that he never dealt drugs. I believe him. At any rate, while Merc was in prison, the principle took over again. His mind initially couldn't accept it. But then, after he got clean and was released, he didn't hang around the same criminal crew. He changed his behavior, and gradually his mind changed.

As he became cleaner and straighter, he started thinking clearer. He subsequently spent years as a motivational speaker, teaching at-risk teens and hardcore incarcerated criminals about the principle. Change your behavior, change your friends, fix your body, fix your life. <u>As you begin to get on the correct course, your mind will follow.</u> Good things will happen.

The moment you commit yourself, good things happen.

Whatever you can do, or dream you can, begin it.

Boldness has genius, power, and magic in it!

— *Goethe, "Prelude at the Theatre," Faust*

It All Comes Down to Pleasure or Pain

We've all heard these ideas before: life's a pursuit of pleasure and an avoidance of pain. *"The secret of success is learning how to use pain and pleasure instead of having pain and pleasure use you. If you do that, you're in control of your life. If you don't, life controls you"* (Robbins, p. 56).

So what do we take pleasure in? I don't know about you, but a lot of stuff that's actually painful (bad for me) has given me pleasure. It's quite a paradox: **what seems pleasurable actually causes pain.**

As I discuss in the Eating chapter, we stuff our faces with great-tasting food (pleasure) that makes us fat, poisons our bodies, and gives us diseases (pain). I got great pleasure from smoking pot in my 20's and am now suffering the pain of a bad memory, not to mention how lazy and stupid it made me back then.

From 1969-71, I was a wild pleasure-seeking maniac, from skipping college classes (immediate pleasure with painful consequences) to drag racing on I-95 in South Florida. Great fun, but painful risks and bad pain from tickets and worse. Very stupid. I'm lucky to be alive. I could have died in a fiery crash. But the foolish 19-year-old me felt immortal, invincible. I just flat out ignored the enormous pain my pointless death would have caused my family and the families of the other fools I was racing who might have died along with me. Crazy.

I needed to learn—and am still waging the battle—that what gives pleasure is not always good for me. The pleasure/pain dichotomy comes with paradoxical attributes. I have to pay attention to what I'm paying attention to. Is this pleasurable activity, thought, or event actually a real pleasure, or pain in disguise? **What happens when the fun is done?**

One excellent technique to reprogram our brains so that we immediately flip the switch on something pleasurable, turning it from good to bad in our minds, is known as Neuro- Associative Conditioning (NAC). Essentially, we can train our brains to seek pleasure and avoid pain through simple reinforcement. Just as we train our brains to turn negative thoughts into positive ones through Mindfulness (See Chapter 3, Equanimity), we should do the same thing with pain and pleasure. You can *"Condition your nervous system to associate pleasure to those things you want to continuously move toward and pain to those things you need to avoid"* (Robbins, p. 112). Robbins spends several chapters developing these ideas and techniques.

We can condition ourselves through simple reinforcement. Every time we recognize that what seems pleasurable is actually painful—e.g., eating the wrong food, being lazy and skipping exercise to watch TV, indulging in too much alcohol or some stupid drug—we should mindfully pause, make a note of it, and engage in positive self-talk. Just tell ourselves how well we're doing. *That was good. I made the right decision. I did the right thing.* Meditate on it, on how you identified the pain disguised as pleasure. You ripped off its phony face and exposed its true ugly nature.

For me, I take great pleasure in this system. I consider anything that stands in the way of my daily self-improvement to be very painful. Using NAC, I reframe, refocus, and re-see all that food I used to eat for pleasure as hunks and chunks and blobs of fat and poison. When I see pizza, fried food, processed meat, nachos, I now see greasy globs of garbage. Rubbish and trash unfit for scavenging raccoons. That might be a bit radical for you, but it works for me.

<u>Persist</u>

I will spend more time in the first **S** (Sustain) discussing this, but it's very self-explanatory. You cannot flag, drag, or sag in your efforts. This must be a daily routine. If you get depressed or distracted, or God forbid, a tragedy knocks you off your schedule, it is even more critical that you get back on your schedule to overcome the depression, distraction, or tragedy. Only by persisting and maintaining your daily schedule will you accomplish your goals.

> *Nothing in the world can take the place of persistence. Talent will not; nothing is more common than unsuccessful men with talent. Genius will not; unrewarded genius is almost a proverb. Education will not; the world is full of educated derelicts. Persistence and determination alone are omnipotent. The slogan 'Press On' has solved and always will solve the problems of the human race.*
>
> —Calvin Coolidge

"Progress Is Our Most Important Product" – General Electric's tagline for decades

Both as a noun and a verb. As a noun, make daily progress. Think about it all day as part of your mantra: am I making progress? Reward yourself with positive self-talk if you are: *"I'm making progress. I'm strong and focused."* Measure your progress in your journal. Record all your progress in everything—your production, plans, writing, diet, exercise, and reading—in every element of being *PEERLESS*. As a verb, keep progressing. March relentlessly forward in your MS toward achieving your daily, weekly, monthly goals.

Production, Purpose, and Progress Killers

Time Wasters The biggest obstacle to your success is you. Very likely, you waste too much time. I know I do. Even now, with my *PEERLESS* system and all my projects, goals, and determination, I still get on SM too much. I still find my attention wavering; I still get unaccountably lazy. Of course, I could say that I'm driving and pushing myself too hard. I sometimes even doubt what I'm doing, despite all the progress I've made. I still lose focus and energy and just wonder if it's all worth it, if I'm deluding myself, if I can really do it. It's the "Lizard Brain" fighting you.

The Lizard Brain

In 1954, the limbic cortex was described by neuroanatomists. Since that time, the limbic system of the brain has been implicated as the seat of emotion, addiction, mood, and lots of other mental and emotional processes. It is the part of the brain that is phylogenetically very primitive. Many people call it the "Lizard Brain," because the limbic system is about all a lizard has for brain function. It is in charge of fight, flight, feeding, fear, freezing up, and fornication. (Troncale)

Don't let your lizard brain run your life. The first step in defeating the lizard brain is to monitor and control how we spend our time every day. An idle brain is the lizard's workshop. When we're engaged in doing things that are of minimal or no importance, we're opening ourselves up to feeling irrational emotions and fears, which can only have a negative effect on our lives.

📖 Record in your journal at night what you did all day. Do that for a week or two to get a good sample size. Be diligent and honest about it. Ask yourself:

❓ What exactly did I do all day? My job, my business, an activity?

❓ What do I do too much of that just wastes time? TV watching? Phone surfing? Social media? Consumed with checking the news? Tim Ferriss advises that we go on a **"low-information diet,"** noting that *"Most information is time-consuming, negative, irrelevant to your goals, and outside of your influence"* (4HWW, p. 87). He notes quite correctly that if anything truly important happens, we'll hear about it.

❓ What can we do to make staying productively busy a daily habit rather than a sporadic burst of intermittent energy where sometimes we do some things, but other times we do as little as possible?

❓ What can we do to make more money, strengthen our brain, our body, our relationships?

❓ How did our Lizard Brains affect us today?

❓ How can we better fight the Lizard Brain tomorrow?

So, what's keeping us from doing all of these things? Why do we waste so much time? What is our main problem?

Ourselves. My main problem is Me. I often think that what I'm doing is too hard, too strict, too rigorous. Why can't I just relax more and let it go? Just stop trying to be so rigid and rough on myself. Just ditch this never-let-up system. I wonder right now, this very minute I'm writing, if I'm pushing myself too hard and if it wouldn't be more fun and wonderful just to let up and let myself go?

But then, I snap back and remind myself that in structure, there is freedom; in a process and plan, there is joy and relaxation. In vacationing from the plan and the process, there is a vacancy. *"Discipline is freedom,"* as Jocko Willink says.

❓

Am I happier, fuller, richer, more fulfilled—anything good at all—when I'm focused and on track and on schedule? YES

- Or was I happier before I got focused, wrote an MS, codified my Goals, came up with a system and a plan? NO

- Was I living a better life not knowing what to do with every day and the rest of my life? Just cruising along, free as a bird? NO

- Was I better off before my *PEERLESS* system? NO. The answer is a resounding NO. I was worse off. Without a doubt.

When we go through personal mental struggles, get weak, and want to give it all up, the only antidote is to get a grip on ourselves by returning to our mantras, come back to our breathing, meditating, mindfulness.

<u>We must continually win the battle with our current selves so that our future selves can enjoy longer, healthier lives.</u>

We can never let up, never stop reminding ourselves of our MS, Goals, and Purpose. Like AA teaches people trying to kick drinking, the battle rages on every single hour of every single day. Hopefully, it's not that bad for you. But for me, even writing this book this very minute (10:50 AM, 8/1/2020), I'm battling myself. Despite all the progress I've made and all of my mantras, determination, and reasons for doing this, the excuses and doubts haunt me. The Lizard Brain wages its self-destructive war.

So, if *you* don't experience such self-doubts and mood swings, if you've got your Lizard Brain under control, then you can definitely do this.

We soldier on.

Now let's talk about eating because we are, indeed, what we eat.

CHAPTER 2

Eating

"Getting your food right is the number one human upgrade."

—Dave Asprey (*Super Human*, p. 41)

We don't have to be "unhealthy" and/or overweight to study and reconsider what we're currently eating. We should first start by discussing our eating habits with our doctors. Generally, our doctor should know if we're unhealthy or overweight. However, there are many charts and resources to help us determine if we're overweight and what our ideal weight is.

> *America is on the wrong track. Two out of every three of us are overweight or obese. Diabetes and high blood pressure are on the rise. Heart attacks, strokes, and cancer are distressingly common. Many factors contribute to these complex problems, but the basic reasons are simple: we eat too much, we choose the wrong foods, and we don't get enough exercise. ("A Guide to Healthy Eating," Harvard Medical School)*

Now, get ready for the truth that may or may not shock you: alas, your doctor may not take the time or even know exactly what to advise you about eating. *You* need to take charge of your health, starting with your eating habits.

As I already briefly mentioned, Dr. William Davis's *Undoctored* is a definitive scathing indictment of the healthcare system. In the book, he makes the disturbing case that the average American doctor knows very little about nutrition and how to prevent diseases by addressing deficiencies, preferring treatment rather than prevention. I'll share more of what he has to say in Chapter 8, but here's a taste that should make you shake your head in disgust:

> *Undoctored wouldn't be necessary if the healthcare system lived up to its name and provided actual "health"—but it does not. It does nothing of the sort,... If healthcare truly provided health, then your primary care doctor would counsel you on correcting common nutritional deficiencies,... If it doesn't involve a prescription, an injection, sedation, a bowel prep, a trip to the hospital, and big fees, health issues such as nutrition and correcting nutritional deficiencies are typically pooh-poohed as meaningless or ineffective by the medical community, or at least not part of their role. The unspoken secret is that providers prefer treatment over prevention, expensive over inexpensive, patent-protectable over non-patent protectable, billable procedure over nonbillable procedure,... (p. 26, 27, & 30)*

That quote alone should make us wary and motivate us to take a more active role in assessing and addressing our healthcare needs.

We'll delve into such assessments, many prevention and treatment alternatives to your doctors, home testing options, crowd-sourcing communities that share information, and truly life-changing over-the-counter (OTC) supplements you've probably never heard of as we progress through the program here. But let's start with the food we eat.

Although not diseases per se, **many of the foods we eat may as well be diseases because they are either disease-ridden themselves or they directly cause diseases.**

The GUT Biome

As Hippocrates knew 2500 years ago, "*All diseases begin in the gut.*" If the food we eat isn't properly digested and processed, all the other systems in our body are in jeopardy of being destroyed.

So how do we ensure that our guts are healthy? By understanding how the food we eat affects our health and by radically adjusting our diets to take care of our "gut buddies," as Dr. Stephen Gundry, in *The Longevity Paradox*, refers to the bacteria living inside us.

Your fate is in the hands of the trillions of bacteria that live inside, on, and around you.... In fact, 90% of "your" cells are not actually human cells at all. They are the cells and bacteria, viruses, fungi, and worms that live on you and inside you, commonly referred to as the microbiome.... (Gundry, p. 4)

> *These bacteria digest our food, remove toxins, fight infections, and produce the vitamins and chemicals essential to keep the body running right.*

Using a brilliant metaphor, Gundry calls our body a condo, us the landlord, and the bacteria our tenants. They live inside of us, and they can keep our condo nice and clean and in tip-top shape only if we do our part by keeping up with their maintenance requests.

Our relationship with our bugs has always been, and continues to be, symbiotic; in other words, their health is dependent on you and vice versa. You take care of them, and they'll take care of you—for the long term....I've seen dramatic reversals of diseases...directly linked to alterations we've made to their gut bacteria. (Gundry, p. 5 & 10)

So what exactly goes wrong with our guts? When the digestive tract lining is not filtering properly due to tears and holes, food particles, bacteria, and toxic waste can pass into our bloodstream. The outward symptoms of this "Leaky Gut Syndrome" include fatigue, constipation, diarrhea, joint pain, weight gain, bloating, and headaches. All of these symptoms are, in turn, caused by chronic inflammation due to that leaky gut, and lead to all the diseases of aging, including diabetes, heart disease, autoimmune diseases, and Alzheimer's. The usual suspects cause a leaky gut: a bad diet high in processed foods, carbs, sugars, trans fats, and not enough fiber. This environment is perfect for the survival and proliferation of lectins—the primary result of the bad diet and the cause of leaky gut.

Lectins are sticky protein molecules that bind to carbohydrates. For plants, lectins are useful to defend them against attacks from fungi, parasites, and mold. But in the human digestive tract, lectins resist being digested by enzymes or broken down by stomach acid. Still intact, they keep doing their job: attaching themselves to our cells, ripping and tearing their way through our stomach lining and intestines, ultimately busting through into our bloodstream. Freely traveling around our bodies, they bind to every tissue they can find, causing inflammation everywhere they go, wreaking havoc on our otherwise good health.

Where do lectins come from? From the food we shouldn't eat and that I'll soon discuss in detail: sugars, grains, beans, peanuts, tomatoes, potatoes, corn, peppers, dairy, processed foods, even eggs and chicken and some seafood.

I hear you thinking: I can't stop eating *all* of those foods just to get rid of lectins. Okay. Your choice. But reducing their amounts, by whatever we can, reduces lectins' numbers as well. Easier to fight a small army than a large army.

"Eliminating Lectins is an important step in healing your gut and slowing (and reversing) the effects of aging," says Dr. Gundry (p. 41).

But lectins aren't our guts' only enemy. Get this: *"nonsteroidal anti-inflammatory drugs (NSAIDs) such as ibuprofen, Aleve, Advil...[are] both the number one pharmaceutical seller and the number one cause of inflammation—the very thing they're meant to treat!"* (Gundry, p. 41). Nice. All those ten thousand ibuprofen pills I've taken in my life didn't *reduce* the deadly inflammation in my body; they actually *increased* it!

As if that's not enough of a backstabbing from Big Pharma, here's another. I've taken acid-reflux medicine—Omeprazole (aka, Prilosec and Prevacid)—for decades. It eliminated acid reflux all right **and** killed off trillions of my gut buddies in the process.

Another class of drugs that is disastrous for your gut is proton pump inhibitors (PPIs) and other stomach acid reducers such as Zantac, Prilosec, Nexium, and Protonix. Stomach acid is important and necessary. It kills off most of the bad bugs you swallow…stomach acid is one of the best defenses against bad bugs getting into you, as one of its main purposes is to kill bacteria….So by using stomach acid blockers, you inadvertently wipe out one of your major defense mechanisms against lectins! (Gundry, p. 42 & 43)

It gets even worse: PPIs "*actually poison your brain's mitochondria…making it impossible for them to produce energy….[And they have also been linked] to chronic kidney disease*" (Gundry, p. 44).

🐞 So what can we do for a healthier gut? Change our diets and don't take NSAIDs or PPIs.

> When I help my patients heal their gut wall and balance their gut buddies, their inflammation levels (which I can measure based on the amount of cytokines in their blood) decrease dramatically, and their bodies rapidly repair the damage…. (Gundry, p. 38)

What's Good to Eat

It's pretty basic: to protect and nourish our gut buddies, we need to eat food that's good for us, not bad for us. It's been said a thousand times, but here's the basic advice from Dr. Sinclair: A longevity diet includes "*eating more vegetables, legumes, and whole grains, while consuming less meat, dairy products, and sugar*" (p. 88). Great advice, with the possible exceptions of whole grains and legumes, which are the subject of intense, vehement disagreement among the nutritional experts. I'll discuss the perceived pros and cons of whole grains shortly.

Organic Only!

Buy and eat *only* organic. The evidence is overwhelming and conclusive: the vast majority of our produce and even meat is poisoned. That's right: poisoned.

> *Greens are commonly sprayed with Glyphosate, the main ingredient in the herbicide Roundup [as is]....much of our conventionally grown produce and the greens that are fed to conventionally raised animals. This means that glysophate is hiding in most products containing corn, other grains, industrial feedlot meat, and animal products like non-organic milk, yogurt, cheese, and so on.* (Asprey, *Super Human*, p. 43)

I'm always reluctant to believe shocking news. A poison is routinely sprayed on almost all of the food we then eat? No way. So, I researched it more and found dozens of corroborating sources. It's not a lie, not an exaggeration, and completely inexplicable yet true.

Kissing the Ground is a brilliant new (2020) documentary on Netflix that makes the convincing case that by healing the world's soil, we can heal both ourselves and the planet. In graphic footage after footage, the *desertification* and toxification of our soil, and thus our food, by pesticides (primarily glyphosate) is 100% undeniably documented.

Here's one more source (out of hundreds) confirming the tragic scope of glyphosate and other harmful chemicals in the food we consume and products we routinely use:

Glyphosate destroys your microbiome....[and also inhibits the body's ability to produce] serotonin, the feel good hormone and thyroid hormone....In addition, there are estrogen-like agents in most of our plastics, cosmetics, preservatives, and sunscreens. Exposure to these agents is linked to obesity, diabetes, and other metabolic diseases... breast and ovarian cancer, thyroid problems, and impaired development of the brain.... (Gundry, pp. 31-32)

Until and unless the use of such killer chemicals is prohibited, our only protection from them is to buy and consume organically grown crops.

Vegetables, Vegetables, Vegetables!

All the hype and cliches and advice are 100% correct. You can't eat anything better than vegetables. (Provided they're organically grown.) Good carbs, minerals, and vitamins. Loaded with polyphenols that activate anti-inflammatory and anti-aging genes that make your cells more powerful and younger.

While cognitive abilities naturally decline with age, eating one serving of leafy green vegetables a day may aid in preserving memory and thinking skills as a person grows older, according to a study by researchers at Rush University Medical Center in Chicago. The study was published in Neurology, the medical journal of the American Academy of Neurology.

"Adding a daily serving of green leafy vegetables to your diet may be a simple way to help promote brain health," said study author Martha Clare Morris, ScD, *a nutritional epidemiologist at Rush. "There continue to be sharp increases in the percentage of people with dementia as the oldest age groups continue to grow in number. Effective strategies to prevent dementia are critically needed."*

The study results suggest that people who ate one serving of green, leafy vegetables had a slower rate of decline on tests of memory and thinking skills than people who rarely or never ate them. The study results also suggest that older adults who ate at least one serving of leafy green vegetables showed an equivalent of being 11 years younger cognitively. ("Daily Leafy Greens")

Pretty convincing. The quote is referring primarily to older people, but the advice is applicable to all age groups. If you want to maximize your chances of good cognitive functioning throughout your life, eat vegetables.

Mushrooms

They're supercharged with health benefits because they're rich in antioxidants, polyphenols, polysaccharides, and polyamines—all beneficial for your immune system and gut (Gundry, pp. 195-196).

Fruit

There's healthy fruit and somewhat unhealthy fruit. The knock-on fruit has a high fructose (sugar) content, which is not good.

Healthy fruit: Avocados, Strawberries, blueberries, raspberries, blackberries, apples, kiwi, lemons.

Not-so-healthy fruit (because of their higher carb and sugar content): bananas, grapes, mangoes, cherries, cranberries, and oranges.

Extra-virgin Olive Oil

Often referred to as a "superfood," olive oil's heart-healthy fats provide a time-released flow of energy to the body, while its polyphenols clear the blood of toxins. The evidence is abundant: olive oil is one of the very best substances you can put in your body.

Many studies of the world's concentrations of the oldest living humans indicate that they all have a high amount of olive oil in their diets.

Consume two tbsp of olive oil daily: Both consuming olive oil and the Mediterranean diet, a diet high in olive oil, are associated with healthy aging. The Sardinians and Ikarians also prove this to be true, so I started adding high-quality olive oil to my salads. (Licalzi)

It's an antioxidant, immune system boosting, anti-inflammatory, cholesterol-lowering, diabetes managing, weight reducing powerhouse.

Dr. Gundry also agrees, famously repeating to all he comes in contact with that the best reason to eat food is to ingest the olive oil you cover it in. He sells a polyphenol-rich olive oil, touting it as the world's best. I'm a believer and a customer, happy to attest that it's a delicious olive oil, and I'm convinced it's doing great things for my body.

Okay, let's say you're sold on it, but how, you might wonder, except by pouring it on salads, do you get it into you? Easy. Add it to a protein shake, a recovery shake, coffee, yogurt—anything. It barely affects the flavor at all. Can't taste it. Not too much, anyway. Or just drink it. The recommended amount is two tablespoons per day. A lot of people just drink a tablespoon for half their daily quota.

Nuts

Most nuts are really good for us. I'm not going into the details—they're readily available online—but trust me that nuts do vary in degrees of healthy attributes. No nuts are "bad" for us, though some are healthy and some may not be.

The good ones: macadamia, pistachio, chestnut, walnut, pecan.

The okay ones: almonds.

The not-so-good ones: peanuts (which are actually legumes) and cashews. Both are high in lectins.

Chicken

We're not going to put chicken on trial because, in general, it's considered to be pretty good for us. A lean meat, it's high in protein and low in fat. Chicken is famous for its many health benefits: building muscles, strengthening bones, reducing stress, and boosting immunity. Alas, some naysayers rightly note that battering and frying chicken can most certainly present health risks, as can the antibiotics injected into them as they're raised. Buying organically-raised chickens and grilling them is your best bet.

What's Debatable to Eat or Not

Eggs

For the prosecution: A study published in the *Journal of Atherosclerosis Research* found that *"because egg yolks are loaded with cholesterol, a known risk factor for coronary artery disease and heart attacks, eating one egg per day was just as bad for your heart as smoking five cigarettes per day"* (Loria).

For the defense: Many compelling voices chime in on the health benefits of eggs. Here's a typical one: *"A large egg contains only 77 calories, with 5 grams of fat and 6 grams of protein with all 9 essential amino acids. Rich in iron, phosphorus, selenium and vitamins A, B12, B2 and B5 (among others). About 113 mg of choline, a very important nutrient for the brain"* (Gunnars).

Verdict on Eggs: Despite a few dissenting voices, the consensus is that 1-2 eggs per day are more beneficial than harmful. But be sure to buy eggs from free-range (not "cage-free") organically raised chickens!

Other Dairy: Milk, Cheese, Butter, etc.

For the Prosecution: Here's a summary of the many arguments against drinking milk and eating dairy of any sort: it's said to be unnatural to drink the milk and eat the products made from the milk (cheese, butter, cream) of another creature. Homo Sapiens didn't start doing it until approximately 7500 years ago. Dairy contains harmful antibiotics and hormones, is highly acidic, high in saturated fat, raises insulin levels, causes inflammation, can cause high blood pressure and cholesterol levels, and can lead to thyroid problems and cancer. Although some studies tout dairy's health benefits, the prosecution claims that many, if not most, have been funded by the dairy industry itself. *"The thing is, quality research costs a lot of money. It costs millions of dollars to support studying the health benefits of dairy as well as marketing these benefits to the public. And those who have the most to gain, i.e., the dairy industry, are the most likely to fund the science behind it"* (Satrazemis).

For the defense: Dairy products are a good source of protein, calcium, vitamin D, and potassium, which helps increase bone formation and density. Many proponents of low-fat dairy claim it's the "healthy" alternative since decreasing the fat cuts calories and cholesterol, while protein, calcium, and most other vitamins and minerals remain high.

However, yet again, regarding the subject of low- vs. high-fat, the "experts" radically disagree. After nine years of research, Nina Teicholz, in her book *The Big Fat Surprise: Why Butter, Meat and Cheese Belong in a Healthy Diet,* concludes that

> *it was a mistake to restrict fat but also that our fear of the saturated fats in animal foods—butter, eggs, and meat—has never been based in solid science. A bias against these foods developed early on and became entrenched, but the evidence mustered in its support never amounted to a convincing case and has since crumbled away...[my] book lays out the scientific case for why our bodies are healthiest on a diet with ample amounts of fat and why this regime necessarily includes meat, eggs, butter, and other animal foods high in saturated fat. (pp. 6-7)*

Verdict on Dairy: Hung jury—there's simply too much conflicting information to reach a definitive position. Once again, you need to do your own homework and determine for yourself what and how much (or how little) dairy (milk, cheese, butter, high-fat, low-fat, etc.) to include in your diet.

Grains

Here's another area of vehement disagreement. We love our bread, pasta, rice, cereal, etc. Few people love bread more than I do. Pasta, rice, and cereal haven't been too hard for me to quit. But bread? It's been the #1 toughest food for me to stop eating. In fact, I "cheat" with bread more than with anything else in my diet. I do so at my own risk, alas.

For the Prosecution: Dr. Davis minces no words in his scathing condemnation of grains (including bread, corn, and rice):

> ...you ought to be terrified by grains.... [and] Once you recognize the extraordinary and disruptive effect of grains... and remove them, extraordinary and unexpected health benefits unfold....to a large degree, I regard the healthcare system...as the system largely created to treat the consequences of grain consumption. (pp. 113 & 122-23)

Almost shocking in its implications, Dr. Davis's position is held by many others. Dr. Gundry warns about grains being high in lectins, raising your triglyceride levels, and causing NASH (fatty liver disease) (p. 108). There's little debate that white, processed grains—bread, rice, pasta—are bad for us. If it's white, that means it's been refined, processed, and stripped of its nutrients. There's just no point in eating it. It's empty carbs and sugars. The bone of contention is with whole grains, those grains that have been less aggressively processed and are closer to their original identity as wheat. Yet, the case against wheat is strong because it has four very shady defendants: gluten, zonulin, glyphosate, and triglycerides.

Gluten is the protein in wheat, and whether or not we have a medically proven intolerance to it, it's not good for us. Research abounds, making a strong case that we should all avoid wheat because of its gluten alone.

Zonulin, the lesser-known second culprit—the brains behind the wheat operation—is sneaky bad for us.

> *Wheat causes inflammation and gastrointestinal distress and contributes to autoimmune disease and a host of other issues by stimulating an over release of zonulin, a protein that controls the permeability of the tight junctions between the cells lining your gut. It does that whether or not you tell yourself that you tolerate wheat just fine. With excess zonulin, the gaps between your intestinal cells open, allowing bacteria, undigested food, and bacterial toxins to flood into your bloodstream....They make you old...They do this no matter what you think about gluten. (Asprey, Super Human, p. 42)*

Glyphosate has already been thoroughly prosecuted and convicted of killing us softly but surely.

So, what about triglycerides? The most common type of body fat, triglycerides, store excess energy, but

> *a high triglyceride level is indicative of health problems. As a guide, your HDL level should be equal to or higher than your triglyceride level, which basically signifies that you're recycling more fat than is being stored.... Grains also raise triglyceride levels... [resulting in] fatty liver disease (NASH)...a condition from eating "healthy" whole-grain goodness and washing it down with fructose-laden juices and fruits. (Gundry, pp. 104-108)*

High Triglycerides also result in fatty buildups within artery walls, increasing the risk of a heart attack or stroke. *"Wheat/grain elimination reduces trigylcerides dramatically..."* (Davis, p. 339).

For the Defense: Nonetheless, despite all the evidence, some people defend whole grain wheat. Many people tout whole grains as being healthy and nutritious because they provide iron, fiber, and vitamins E and B, as well as some effective antioxidants. They're a rich source of good carbs, proteins, and unsaturated (good) fat. Besides whole grain, rye bread is noted for having less gluten, while sourdough is promoted for its low GI (glycemic index) content. However, despite the positives, most advocacy for grains is lukewarm at best. Typical among the many concluding statements regarding grains is this: *"Foods made from whole grain are also better for you..."* (*Transcend*, p. 214). Note the *"better for you"*; not *"good for you,"* just *"better."* Why? Because whole grain, when compared to white processed grain, *is "better* for you."

If it's organic, that removes glyphosate from the scene of the crime. Dave's Bread is excellent in that regard. It comes in several organic varieties of whole grain. Very tasty and high quality. But it still has gluten, zonulin, and triglycerides. If you want to risk it, moderation may get you by.

Verdict on Grains: It's a split decision, but not a hung jury: wheat is guilty as charged. It does more harm than good, and it could lead to your premature death.

Animal Protein/Fat; aka, Meat

Red Meat

A VERY sore subject with highly contentious opposing views. We've all heard that *everything in moderation* is a good rule of thumb. But is that so with red meat? It depends on which "experts" you favor. Most argue that it's a direct cause of heart attacks since it contains more cholesterol and saturated fats than other sources of protein. Some argue the opposite.

For the prosecution: I could call thousands of witnesses, but I'll just call three.

Dr. Sinclair:

> *Study after study has demonstrated that heavily animal-based diets are associated with high cardiovascular mortality and cancer risk. Processed red meats are especially bad. Hotdogs, sausage, ham, and bacon might be gloriously delicious, but they're ingloriously carcinogenic, according to hundreds of studies that have demonstrated a link between these foods and colorectal, pancreatic, and prostate cancer. (p. 99)*

Dr. Gundry:

> *Conventionally raised livestock are fed antibiotics in shocking quantities... Killing off the gut buddies that keep you lean and flexible well into your old age. In fact, obesity in humans is marked by a decrease in bacterial diversity in the gut... [Furthermore] animal protein causes dangerous inflammation, which is an utter disaster for longevity....And a diet high in animal fat inhibits our natural defense mechanisms against cancer cells. (Gundry, pp. 30-31, 100, & 115)*

Dave Asprey:

> *When you eat a diet high in animal protein, you can expect a 75% increased risk of dying from all causes over 18 years, a 400% increase risk of dying of cancer, and a 500% increase risk of diabetes compared to someone who restricts his or her animal proteins....Restricting protein intake also helps to boost autophagy, your all important cellular recycling program. (Asprey, Super Human, p. 47 & 48)*

For the Defense: The meat industry. As you might expect, they have their own set of studies that claim to prove eating meat does no harm. In fact, it does a body good.

Assorted freelance writers for bodybuilding and various men's magazines, very few of them MDs from my research, stress that humans are carnivores (actually omnivores), meat is good for your bones, muscles, and energy, and the anti-meat argument is a myth and a lie. Many of these articles conclude by saying it tastes great! *"So be true to your human nature and to your taste buds. Don't cut meat out of your life"* (Araki). *"Finally and most importantly, meat makes the food much tastier and satisfying. There is also a large variety of meat preparations and dishes that give us better pleasures of dining"* (Collins).

However, just when the case seems lost, the defense calls two star witnesses (from among quite a few others, I might add but don't for purposes of con-ciseness and brevity).

As we've already briefly discussed, Dr. Davis, who rips to shreds the entire healthcare system, also demolishes many of the USFDA's formerly sacro-sanct dietary guidelines. Davis convincingly argues that not only is red meat *not* the killer the prosecution claims it to be, but it's also actually an essential, natural, and *healthy* choice for people to eat.

Davis argues that based on studying what *Homo Sapiens* have eaten through-out history, it's natural and best to eat animal fat and protein because that's what we've adapted to eating: *"...meat consumption is therefore programmed into a digestive health, now causing us to be reliant on nutrients from the source"* (Davis, p. 127). We need what meat provides:

> *Fats, unlike carbohydrates, are essential, as necessary as water or oxygen.... consuming the fat of animals is also part of our natural physiology.... Yet we've been told over the last 50 years that fats, especially animal fats, are the worst for health....[but] limiting fat consumption was a mistake we made starting 50 years ago, a man-made blunder based on misinterpretation, misrepresentation, the leanings of dietary zealots, and politics. (Davis, p. 129)*

The important distinction must be made between primarily unprocessed red meat—steaks and ground beef—and highly processed lunch meats, bacon, sausage, and hot dogs. Davis claims that

> There are no clinical trials demonstrating that limiting fat or saturated fat provides any health benefits or reduces cardiovascular risk. Likewise, red meat consumption has no relationship to cardiovascular risk if the effects of cured processed meats (salami, sausage, lunch meat, hotdogs) are factored out. (Davis, p. 130)

If true, that's game-changing information: only *processed* meat with its high amounts of sodium and sugar, and its claims to be "healthy" because it's "low-fat" are the killers. Your steak and hamburger are innocent bystanders, framed by the establishment to take the fall so that the real criminals go scot-free.

The supposition is that studies of heart attack and cancer victims have lumped all meat into the equation. That is most people who suffer from diseases linked to eating meat eat *both* unprocessed and processed meat. There has been no consideration given to or even a way to determine whether the cancer and heart disease was caused by a certain meat or all meat. Dr. Davis contends that only processed meat causes diseases.

Dr. Davis doubles down in his closing arguments:

> ...the fats humans are adapted to consuming are the components of animal fat: monounsaturates, saturates, and some polyunsaturates....Fats are satiating.... Don't buy lean cuts of meat; buy fatty cuts. If you eat a steak, eat the fat.... If weight loss is among your goals, one especially powerful strategy is to purposefully load up on fats to induce satiety, thereby reducing your desire to take in more calories.... Taking in healthy fats and oils is liberating, does not promote cardiovascular disease, and helps you break the bonds

of greens and sugars. Of the 6000 generations that Homo Sapiens have walked on this planet, we made the low fat mistake no more than two generations ago. (Davis, p. 132)

Nina Teicholz agrees with Dr. Davis that there is no solid evidence whatsoever to condemn red meat. In fact, she concludes that those who eat animal fat, a.k.a. saturated fat, are healthier than those who do not eat it.

The case against saturated fat has collapsed. Moreover, we now know that there are many good reasons to eat animal foods like red meat, cheese, eggs, and whole milk: they are particularly dense in nutrients....They contain fat and protein in the proportion that humans need. They have been shown to provide the best possible nutrition for healthy growth and reproduction.... And saturated fats, like all fats, do not make people fat....Meat is the central food throughout all of human history, as recorded by humans themselves. We've forgotten our history at our peril. (pp. 334 & 336)

Verdict on Red Meat: Thanks largely to the compelling testimony of Davis and Tiecholz, the jury acquits unprocessed meat, but convicts the processed culprits. Despite a strong case against all red meat, their arguments in favor of eating unprocessed meat have planted just enough reasonable doubt in our minds to set unprocessed meat (from grass-fed cows) free. It just might be safe and even healthy to eat high-fat, unprocessed meat. But the low-fat processed stuff will almost certainly lead to diseases. More research and studies are necessary to understand better how that crucial distinction impacts our health and longevity.

Pork

Since we've already put red meat on trial, you can refer to many of the same prosecutorial points to build the case against pork (ham, bacon, sausage): they lead to a variety of diseases because they're high in bad fat and cholesterol, and severely processed from pigs raised on antibiotics that remain in the meat. As with red meat, if you want to eat some in moderation, you might get away with it. Be sure to seek out pork from organically raised pigs if you can find it. But beware of bacon. Although it has its defenders (including Davis and Tiecholz), bacon is very likely the worst meat you can eat. It pains me to say that because no one on earth likes bacon more than I do. Giving it up kills me. Or, more likely, *keeps it* from killing *me*. Not only is it highly processed—and therefore automatically bad news—bacon is loaded with sodium nitrate, a preservative like trans fat that, when cooked becomes extremely toxic. The fact that it's high in saturated fat, as we've already touched on, may or may not be a bad thing, depending on which side of the debate you agree with.

Non-Animal Protein

Legumes

It's a mixed bag at best with legumes, which are all beans, lentils, peas, chickpeas, and peanuts. High in protein and fiber, they're also high in carbs. They have a high concentration of lectins, that we've already prosecuted for preventing the absorption of nutrients, causing inflammation, and being toxic to your cells and nerves. However, some argue that lectins are neutralized when cooked. That's debatable. Regardless, watch out for the popular raw peanut, with all of its lectins intact. And all legumes, cooked or not, contain protease inhibitors and saponins that can cause leaky gut. Legumes attack our intestinal walls, creating tears and fissures that allow bacteria and other toxins to pass into the bloodstream. Not good. Eat legumes at your own risk.

All the Other Stuff

High Carbs & Sugars

Although the facts about carbs and sugars are debated endlessly, they are two potentially lethal bullets to avoid if you want to lose weight and be healthier. Despite heated disagreement, the consensus is that *"the typical modern diet is now weighted so heavily toward carbohydrates, and in particular, refined sugars and starches, that it's literally killing us"* (*Transcend,* p. 211).

There are "good" carbs and sugars and "bad" carbs and sugars. "Good" carbs take time to break down into glucose, but "bad" carbs quickly turn to glucose, causing a spike in blood sugar.

Good carbs include whole grain bread, brown rice, and beans (though the merits of all of those foods are highly questionable, as we've already discussed), and vegetables (the only food beyond reproach—as long as they're organic).

Bad carbs are anything refined, processed, and primarily white (and/or grains): bread (yes, hamburger and hot dog buns), pasta, tortillas, potatoes (yes, french fries too), rice, cereal (yes, *all* breakfast cereal), and fried foods with breading (yes, fried chicken too). Eliminating those foods *"is the single most important thing you can do to reduce risk of metabolic syndrome and type 2 diabetes...[and] excess weight"* (*Transcend,* p. 213*).*

As you can no doubt tell from this and many of my other preceding attempts at analyzing the conflicting information, it can be very confusing to sort through the "experts'" opinions about carbs, and most other food-related issues.

Here's one fairly informative and balanced article on carbs to get you started: https://www.webmd.com/food-recipes/features/carbohydrates#1.

Sugars

Although sugar gets a bad rap—mostly deserved—the fact is, we'd die very quickly without sugar. Our cells depend on sugar as their primary source of energy. For most of us, the carbs we eat are a sufficient source of sugar. If we eat any pasta, fruit juices, dairy products (milk, butter, cream, cheese), or high-starch vegetables (potatoes, corn, etc.), we're getting plenty of sugar for our cells. What we don't need is the extra sugar sources from soft drinks, candy, pastries, and ice cream, etc. As with so many other substances we eat, the experts don't always agree. Dr. Gundry says that sugar *"is an absolute disaster for health and longevity"* (p. 33). Yet, Dr. Fossel concludes his discussion of sugar by asking, *"Is sugar* really *all that bad? Again, it's a matter of context"* (p. 167).

Fats

As discussed regarding dairy and meat, there's vehement disagreement regarding fat. In *Eat Fat, Get Thin*, Dr. Mark Hyman details a diet program based on scientific evidence supporting the importance of fat in weight loss and overall health. *"What is the single best thing you can do for your health, weight, and longevity? Eat more fat! That's right. Eat more fat to lose weight; feel good; prevent heart disease, diabetes, dementia, and cancer; and live longer"* (p. 3).

Dr. Davis also weighs in: *"There are no clinical trials demonstrating that limiting fat or saturated fat provides any health benefits or reduces cardio-vascular risk"* (p. 130).

The best advice I can give is the usual—do your due diligence and make your own decision. But, definitely read the food labels and follow this simple advice: Unsaturated fat *may* be safe. Saturated fats may or may not be safe, though Tiecholz encourages us to eat them, saying the case against them *"has collapsed"* (p. 334). Yet, it's worth noting Dr. Gundry's warning that saturated fats cause inflammation that *"sparks hunger"* (p. 212). Trans fats are definitely unsafe in any amount.

 and **Clearly—if anything at all is clear about food—we have to do our own due diligence and arrive at our own conclusions.**

What's Definitely Bad to Eat

Vegetable Oils (Corn, Soy, Canola)

Terrible for us, they're chemically unstable, promoting the formation of free radicals that directly damage our DNA, *"having effects similar to those of radiation"* (Asprey, *Game Changers*, p. 182). Typically high in trans fats, they clog our arteries and lead to strokes, heart attacks, cancer, diabetes, and obesity. They cause general inflammation, which exacerbates and accelerates all other health problems. They're also generally contaminated with pesticides and depleted of minerals and vitamins, besides containing MSG and lots of salt. Killers, any way you look at them.

Fried Foods

It's all about the vegetable oil and the process of frying. As if that's not bad enough, fried foods have almost zero nutritional value because when proteins are fried, they are dissipated and turn into a carcinogen, acrolein. Bad stuff.

Processed Foods

According to the Academy of Nutrition and Dietetics, a "processed" food is any food that's been changed before you eat it.

> *Processed foods are land mines of sugar, high fructose corn syrup, wheat and corn, hydrogenated oils, sodium nitrate, herbicide and pesticide residues, genetically modified ingredients with Bt toxin and glyphosate, bovine growth hormone, antibiotic residues, acrylamides, aspartame, synthetic food coloring, even arsenic. (Davis, p. 141)*

The "processing" of foods often involves using trans-fatty oils, stripping away nutrients, and adding chemical preservatives, salt, and sugar, which translates to more toxins and calories and, therefore, more harm to our bodies.

Many studies have proven as much, including a recent one published in *The American Journal of Clinical Nutrition* that found that telomeres are shortened by eating ultra-processed foods (UPF), and cells age faster. *"Those participants with the highest UPF consumption had almost twice the odds of having short telomeres compared with those with the lowest consumption"*

(Alonso-Pedrero). As I discuss more in Chapter 8, shortened telomeres have been conclusively linked to a higher incidence of numerous diseases, including diabetes, heart disease, hypertension, depression, obesity, and many others. Furthermore, the study also found that people who ate a lot of UPF also, quite logically (since they fill themselves up on UPF), consume less protein, vegetables, and other micronutrients. Instead, they engorge saturated and trans fats, salt, sugar, processed meats, "junk food," and fast food. It's a vicious cycle. The clear conclusion is that UPF is addictive due to its high carbs, sugars, salts, and "great taste": the more you eat UPFs, the more of them you want to eat.

📖 Instead, choose vegetables and other foods that come straight from the organic farm or grass-fed cattle if you choose to eat some meat.

📖 Read the labels: avoid packaged foods with lots of chemicals added. That means they've been processed. And that's definitely not a good thing for your health.

Diets

It's worth noting that we should evaluate and pay attention to when and why we're eating. Make sure that we're really hungry for food. Lots of times, people simply eat when they feel empty, not hungry. Is there a psychological reason why you feel empty and, thus, are eating too much or the wrong food? Could be.

At any rate, if we're overweight, we need to lose weight. Period.

The fundamental reason for losing weight is that restricting our calories *"has the potential of significantly extending human life"* (Fossel, p. 12).

I'll discuss a few of the main diets, but if you have one that you like and you think it will work for you, that's fine. But whatever diet you choose, the consensus from the experts is that a low carb and low or no sugar diet is the best. I personally have found that the Mediterranean (sans grain) in combination with Weight Watchers (WW) works very well for a lot of reasons I'll discuss.

When I was overweight, I often felt witless and helpless. I could hardly get out of bed in the morning. The last straw was when I tried to bend over and tie my shoes on 2/4/20. I couldn't do it. I lost my breath, couldn't breathe, and nearly passed out. I sat heavily, nearly collapsing on my bed, to get my breath back. That was it. I knew I was at rock bottom. On that very day, at that very moment, I resolved to change my life.

? Have you hit rock bottom yet? Maybe you don't need to. Maybe you're not in bad shape, physically or mentally, but if you are, don't wait another minute. Start getting healthy and losing weight.

Meal Delivery

Your first and maybe easiest choice is a diet with meals delivered to you: South Beach, Nutrisystem, Hello Fresh, Freshly, Noom, Diet to Go, and many more. I can't really comment on these beyond saying I tried South Beach, and the food is not good. I'm being kind. It was mainly bad. Just terrible. Inedible much of it. I hear Nutrisystem food is better, and the ones you prepare yourself can be pretty good.

But I ask this simple question: Why? Why do you have to have food processed in some factory, packed in dry ice, shipped to you, and left at your front door? Why do that when you can go to your local grocery store or health food market and buy it fresh?

That's two main points right there: buy fresh, organic food as much as possible, and prepare it yourself.

I've never liked cooking. It's been a big hurdle for me. I've eaten 80-90% of all my meals in my adult life in restaurants. That's the truth. That is up until 2/4/20, when I changed my ways. It's been rough, I won't lie. If *you* like to shop for food and prepare it yourself, great. You have a big advantage. But if you don't, well, you're going to need to learn to like it. Or at least just do it whether you like it or not.

The delivered meals—however convenient they may be—are *not* fresh, despite what they may claim, likely *not* organic, definitely processed, and expensive to boot.

Furthermore, delivered, pre-packaged meals are just another easy-way-out, path-of-least-resistance shortcut.

The best and really the only effective way to eat healthily and get our bodies right is to do it yourself (DIY). Take extreme ownership of what we eat. Learn all about it—the right foods, the right preparations, the right amounts, the right caloric restriction—and DIY.

Like everything else in this PEERLESS program, we've got to develop the mindset of DIY. The greater the role we play personally in everything, the greater the chances for success. It's all on us. We have to own it.

Ultimately, let's visualize what went on with that food dropped on our doorstep by the UPS guy. Do we really want to trust some company to decide what food we eat in their processed, packaged, shipped to our door meal? The more you actually think about it, the more disgusting it should be to you. Who knows who handled it and where and exactly how this food got from the farm or ranch, to the factory or their own "kitchen" and to you! Visualize that food from its source to you. Too many steps, too many human hands, too many possibilities for corruption and tainting and ruining it.

So, meal plan delivered-to-you food is out. For me, anyway.

My plan—and how I've lost 45 pounds (248-203 right now on 9/17/20 as I write this)—has been a combination of the Mediterranean diet and Weight Watchers.

Mediterranean Diet (MD)

My cardiologist recommends this diet. I have a cardiologist because I had two minor heart attacks in 2005. Tough time with lots of stress. My own fault. I take full responsibility for those heart attacks. Anyway, my heart's okay now and has been for 12 years or so. It's even better since I've lost all that weight.

Very simply, the MD is generally considered to be a very "common sense" diet. Low carbs, no sugars, very little dairy or red meat, fish, lots of vegetables, whole grains, beans, nuts, and olive oil. I'm on board with it except for two objections: 1) Whole grains and beans? We've already discussed the solid case against grains of any sort, and beans don't fare much better when scrutinized. 2) *Bias Alert*: I have to tell you again that I'm sold on the argument and logic presented by Dr. Davis and Nina Tiecholz (among many others) that humans have adapted to and rely on the high fat intake of unprocessed red meat. So lumping all red meat together and saying we shouldn't eat it? That just no longer sits well with me. But, aside from that, the rest of the MD diet is basic, sound advice.

Weight Watchers (WW)

Not actually a "diet"—more of an organized system to *manage* your diet— WW starts with you choosing a diet of some sort and plugging it into their system. WW sets your daily caloric intake and converts all food—every last thing you eat right down to a pinch of pepper, a sprig of parsley, and a few nuts—into its point value. Your daily point limit must not be exceeded or you won't lose weight. Simple as that. For what it's worth, my GP recommends WW. I think he's right to do so. As I said, I loosely follow the MD in selecting what foods will play this point game with me.

FYI: I don't have any stake whatsoever in WW. They only know me as a quarterly subscriber, one of millions. I have nothing to gain by recommending WW except that I do believe it works. It's worked for me, anyway.

The WW point system lets you know how much of your daily allowance of food is used up by every single thing you eat. Let's say you have a salad. You learn to choose olive oil and vinegar dressing rather than ranch or blue cheese because you'll save 3 points. Earlier, you had a 2 point yogurt rather than a 6 point yogurt. And on that yogurt, you only put a pinch of grain-free granola, saving another 2 points. And right there, with those three examples and choices, you've saved 6 points. Good stuff! Very informational, educational, and accountable. You can then later "spend" those 6 points on a delicious snack or dessert if you want. Atkins makes a tasty 6-point, chocolate caramel almond protein bar that could be a good last thing to eat for the day.

Keto

Very popular right now, it's short for ketogenic: it forces the body into using primarily fat for energy instead of carbohydrates; with low carb levels, fats are converted into ketones to fuel the body.

Pros: You can lose weight fast by eating whatever you want except carbs: no bread, pasta, potatoes, etc. Lots of fruits and non-starchy vegetables. All dairy products are allowed, including butter, cream, cheese, and full-fat milk. All meats are allowed.

Cons: For a lot of people, it comes with some harmful side effects: nausea, constipation, diarrhea, headaches, and no energy. Worse than that, it allows and even encourages most processed foods, praising bacon, sausage, butter, and cheese, which are widely regarded as unhealthy.

Verdict? Your call. You be the judge and jury.

Atkins

I call it Keto-Lite. Like Keto, Atkins emphasizes weight loss by burning fat and restricting carbs. But unlike Keto, Atkins allows you to gradually increase your carb intake in phases after you've lost weight. I'm not sure of the point of being on the Atkins diet regime of low carbs and then essentially getting off the low carb plan. There seems to be a roller-coaster of lose, gain, lose, gain built-in. If you're going to get carbs out of your diet and you want to keep the weight off that you worked so hard to lose, just stick with it. The consensus of diet evaluators agrees with me: if you're going low-carb, and you don't care about the health risks of processed food, then go Keto over Atkins.

🔹 If you don't want to join WW or another specific diet pro-gram—or even if you do—The Harvard Medical School is an excellent, concise, no-nonsense resource for all things related to good health. Check out their *"Guide to Healthy Eating"*: https://www.health.harvard.edu/promotions/harvard-health-publications/healthy-eating-a-guide-to-the-new-nutrition?mode=order.

🔹 There are literally dozens of other diets, many just slight variations of one another. Harvard Health also has a good publication that evaluates most of them. You can find *The Diet Review: 39 popular nutrition and weight-loss plans and the science behind them* at https://www.health.harvard.edu/promotions/harvard-health-publications/diet-review.

🔹 Thousands of other books, articles, and websites can teach you in exhaustive detail about what to eat and not eat, carbs, sugars, diets, and thousands of nutritional tips and facts. Just to name one, I recommend the lengthy chapter on Nutrition (pp. 207-312) in *Transcend*.

What Should You Be Drinking?

Water

Lots and lots of water. No doubt you've heard that our bodies are 70% water, just as the planet is 70% water. That should tell us something: we're creatures of the water planet. Fresh water going in flushes your body of toxins.

> *Providing necessary fluids immediately upon waking will jump start your body functions – circulation, respiration, brain function and digestion – all of which require the*

life-sustaining power of water.... It's good for your digestive health, flush[ing] toxins from your stomach, liver, bowels and kidneys....Water minimizes uric acid in the kidneys and promotes bile production in the liver....Staying properly hydrated also keeps your stools from hardening which avoids constipation while ensuring regular evacuation of the toxic matter in your bowels....[It's also good for your] heart health [because] another side effect of uric acid build up is it causes platelets in your blood to accumulate plaque on your arterial walls. Atherosclerosis is one of the primary causes of heart attack since the plaque buildup reduces blood flow to the heart....[Furthermore] by increasing hydration, you not only give your body what it needs in fluids, you also feel more full and tend to eat less. [You'll also have increased energy because when] blood production and flow is better, nutrients are broken down more effectively and both fuel and oxygen get to your cells faster. [Water also assists in] disease prevention. According to the "Journal of the American College of Nutrition," dehydration worsens existing diseases such as asthma, heart disease, dental disease, diabetes and glaucoma. It is even considered a contributing factor to prolonged labor and urinary tract problems. Severe dehydration can lead to organ failure in the brain, heart or kidneys and causes the skin to look older and more sunken. ("The Benefits")

That's quite an exhaustive, convincing list of the benefits of water!

<u>Don't drink your calories!</u>

Avoid milk (including soy milk), milkshakes, all sodas, sugary liquids, fruit juices, and any highly processed drinks, such as energy drinks and sports drinks. They're loaded with sugar and likely other toxins.

<u>Alcohol</u>

For weight loss, red wines are okay, but not white wines or beer, with the exception of Bud Light—which is brewed from rice—and a few artisan brands. As for spirits, vodka and gin ain't bad! Again, a simple Google search will turn up lots of info for you should you like to drink and want to minimize its harm to your health.

Protein Shakes

A great way to get 30 grams of your daily protein—and lose weight—is to drink a protein shake in the morning. Tim Ferriss reports that his father's monthly weight-loss tripled when he drank the 30-gram protein shake instead of when he didn't (*4HB*, p. 95). Tim also recommends Ascent Native Fuel Whey Protein powder. Of course, there are many good protein powder brands in many flavors, but the consensus seems that Whey is preferable. I say this because there is a debate among the "experts." I'm biased toward and 100% sold on Tim Ferriss, so I'm going with his recommendations on most things. Of course, I do my research and look for conflicting viewpoints. But when there is no compelling opposition to what Ferriss says, I trust him.

<u>BTW, how much protein do you need?</u>

I used this handy calculator to determine that I *need* 74 grams per day: https://globalrph.com/medcalcs/protein-requirements-daily/. BUT, as I discuss in the chapter on Exercise, if you want to lose the bad weight (fat) while gaining muscle, you should up your protein intake to 1 or even 1.5 grams for every pound of body weight. So, since I weigh 205, I should have 200-300 grams of protein a day. I'm currently up to 130-150 a day and monitoring how I feel. The trick is to get more protein without getting too many calories. As I said, I'll discuss that more later.

Coffee

Bias alert: I love coffee. But I didn't until 7 or 8 years ago. Probably had less than 5 cups of coffee my entire life until I turned 62 or 63. Then, suddenly, I discovered iced coffee. I live in Florida and just don't care for hot liquids. I like my tea iced, my water loaded with ice cubes, and my beer—when I have one—nearly frozen. I start my day with glass after glass of ice-cold water, punctuated by a 16 oz. Yeti tumbler of iced coffee. Within 15 minutes or less, I'm wide awake, energetic, enthusiastic, mindful, fired up...you name it, I'm it. Rip roarin' into my day!

The experts debate heatedly over coffee's pros and cons. I'm going to ignore the cons and just tell you the pros. Just kidding. But seriously, the pros are pretty convincing.

> *Two 2017 studies published in the annals of internal medicine correlate coffee drinking with a longer lifespan. A large European study found that those participants who drank the most coffee had a 10% lower risk of dying from any cause compared to those who didn't drink any coffee at all.* (Peters, p. 80)

> *The results of a study conducted by Professor Kjeld Hermansen of Aarhus University's Department of Clinical Medicine concluded that a moderate intake of coffee can have a health-promoting effect. An intake of three to four cups a day is associated with: A 25-percent reduction in the risk of developing type 2 diabetes and Parkinson's disease. A 10-percent reduction in the risk of apoplexy. A beneficial effect on Alzheimer's disease and depression.....[However], anxiety sufferers, pregnant women and those who consume insufficient amounts of calcium should be careful with their coffee consumption.* (Persson)

> *...newer studies [have] found a possible association between coffee and decreased mortality. Coffee may offer some protection against:*

> * *Parkinson's disease*

- *Type 2 diabetes*

- *Liver disease, including liver cancer*

- *Heart attack and stroke*

Coffee still has potential risks, mostly due to its high caffeine content. For example, it can temporarily raise blood pressure. Women who are pregnant, trying to become pregnant or breastfeeding need to be cautious about caffeine. High intake of boiled, unfiltered coffee has been associated with mild increase in cholesterol levels.

The bottom line? Your coffee habit is probably fine and may even have some benefits. But if you have side effects from coffee, such as heartburn, nervousness or insomnia, consider cutting back. (Hensrud)

Intermittent Fasting (IF)

Dr. Sinclair extols the benefits of IF: **"If there is one piece of advice I can offer, one sure-fire way to stay healthy longer, one thing you can do to maximize your lifespan right now, it's this: eat less often"** *[bold is mine for emphasis]* (p. 89). Eat. Less. Often. His #1 piece of advice. Such strong advice should really sink in and be taken.

Dave Asprey agrees: *"it's one of the most painless high impact ways to live longer"* (*Super Human*, p. 49).

I'm a big believer in just eating in a 4-hour window during the day. It's not for everybody, and it took me a few months to get used to it, but I don't eat anything until 3:00 at the earliest. I try to go until 5:00 if possible. Then, I eat my favorite eggs, fruit bowl, and toast meal (cheating a bit to have some thin gluten-free toasted bread), or a huge salad, or a bowl of vegetarian chili, or a high-fat steak and some grilled vegetables, or any number of other meals. If I'm hungry later, I might have some fresh blueberries and strawberries in a low-fat, no sugar yogurt at around 7:30. Or a protein shake or some nuts or perhaps a protein bar. Then, I'm done. I make sure I don't eat anything else. In that way, I've fasted for 19-21 hours every day, depending on how late in the day I first eat.

IF will definitely help you lose weight because when the hunger pains hit, you know that your body's eating itself—burning fat and even more than that. The following compelling information is from this article: https://www.hopkinsmedicine.org/health/wellness-and-prevention/ intermittent-fasting-what-is-it-and-how-does-it-work.

IF has a lot more health benefits than just helping you lose weight:

> *Dr. Mark Mattson, a Johns Hopkins neuroscientist who has studied intermittent fasting for 25 years, says that our bodies have evolved to be able to go without food for many hours, or even several days or longer. "When changes occur with this metabolic switch, it affects the body and brain." One of Mattson's studies published in the New England Journal of Medicine revealed data about a range of health benefits associated with the practice. These include a longer life, a leaner body and a sharper mind. "Many things happen during intermittent fasting that can protect organs against chronic diseases like type 2 diabetes, heart disease, age-related neurodegenerative disorders, even inflammatory bowel disease and many cancers," he says.*
>
> *Here are some intermittent fasting benefits research has revealed so far:*
>
> - ***Thinking and memory**. Studies discovered that intermittent fasting boosts working memory in animals and verbal memory in adult humans.*
>
> - ***Heart health**. Intermittent fasting improved blood pressure and resting heart rates as well as other heart-related measurements.*

- **Physical performance.** *Young men who fasted for 16 hours showed fat loss while maintaining muscle mass. Mice who were fed on alternate days showed better endurance in running.*

- **Diabetes and obesity.** *In animal studies, intermittent fasting prevented obesity. And in six brief studies, obese adult humans lost weight through intermittent fasting.*

- **Tissue health.** *In animals, intermittent fasting reduced tissue damage in surgery and improved results.*

That's a convincing case for IF, don't you think?

Okay, so how can we stick with the whole eating better, being on a diet regimen?

Think pleasure vs. pain. Ask yourself: How much total time do you spend eating during the day? What is the actual time you are putting food into your mouth and chewing it? Is it 60 minutes? 90 minutes? Let's just say that you're eating for 1.5 hours every day.

If we're overweight, we've likely been eating food that we enjoy eating. Fried foods, pasta, burgers, fries, pizza, ribs, nachos, chips, cake, cookies, ice cream, and drinking beer and soda. You know what you eat. High in carbs, calories, and sugars. Bad stuff. But it tastes so good! We love the taste of our food. It gives us pleasure.

So for an hour and a half of pleasure a day, we are suffering the pain 24/7/365 of what it is doing to our bodies. After we finish those ribs, that pizza, that 6-pack, that bowl of ice cream, or a candy bar, what's next? Another candy bar? A bag of chips? Your other favorite meal or snack, whatever it may be? I'll tell you what's really next: our body is very unhappy with us. It has to digest and process that poison, and we will get fatter from having eaten it.

What we need to do is tell ourselves that this brief fleeting moment of an hour and a half a day of having pleasure is not worth the lifelong pain. Do we really want this pleasure that badly? We are causing such harm to our bodies and our lives because we cannot give up this pleasure.

Here are some journal entries of mine when I first started my diet:

Feb 3/2020: Started WEIGHT WATCHERS!

Weight Watchers/South Beach:

- *Must lose weight*

- *Knees, back, out of breath, look and feel terrible, can't hardly move, aging faster and worse than I ever thought possible in my worst-case scenarios,*

- *The sugar and carbs and calories must go*

- *Must lose 30 pounds minimum*

- *You are what you eat is so true...arthritis, pain everywhere, no energy, bad sleep, total body breakdown...yet it's more important to eat the way I eat than to look, feel, and be better in 100 ways...*

- *I'm literally killing myself with the food I eat and the weight I'm carrying*

- *TIME TO REVERSE COURSE NOW, FEB. 4, 2020...*

- *Now I have this non-stop ache in my left cheek running down my left leg....maybe that's what finally prompted me to stop...change...*

- *I MUST BE STRONG AND DO IT...*

Day 1: smooth and good start

Day 2: same...already noticing my system feeling better

Day 3: only used 28, not 32 points...didn't eat until 3:00...intermittent fasting + south beach food is a big part of my WW diet

Day 4: not even hungry! Almost Noon and haven't eaten...feeling very optimistic and determined...

Day 5: good

Day 6: a mantra I've been repeating: pleasure/pain.

Day 8: Been hitting something of a wall the past 3 days. Body and mind resisting. Feeling weaker. More hungry. More tempted to eat a big meal. I won't. I'll fight through it, but it's tough. Kind of headachy and lightheaded. Symptom of my body eating itself, feeding off the stored fat to get by. Good. Gotta reprogram the signals from my mind and body into positives rather than negatives. Hunger feels good. Love that weak feeling. The weaker I feel, the stronger I'm getting. I'll eat in 2-3 hours from now.

Day 9: Pathetic how weak and stupid I could be in prioritizing and choosing EATING over HEALTH. Bizarre how weak humans can be. How insane, really. How could I have been so addicted to food!!! That's what it boils down to: A FOOD ADDICTION!!! I could not stop eating whatever I wanted. I chose to deal with all the horrible effects of eating rather than stop eating! Hard to logically and rationally understand it. Addiction makes us insane. Doing great. Feeling better than I have in years.

Day 22: Feb 26, 2020: Slipped last night and ate a lot of mixed nuts. They always bother me in the middle of the night too. Feel bloated and slightly off. Gotta cut down to nuts only in the day and only a few. This WW losing weight is slow going. Tough grind. Really craved a burger and fries last night...and candy/cookies...but fought through it...

Some good days, some bad. Progress, setbacks, regroup, try again. Left foot, right foot. We soldier on. And I hadn't even started *PEERLESS* or writing this book. That was still 5 months away! Progress is slow and incremental, but once on track, progress, plans, productivity gather momentum and tend to snowball into even more and greater things.

Now, here's my entry today:

Day 195 Monday August 17, 2020

BACK TO SCHOOL FOR LUKE!!!!!!!!!

> *Weigh 209. Goal for this week, get down to 206 by next Monday. More IT, keep under my points, and just be hungry. Reading and writing a LOT. Sustaining and meditating and just feeling damn good. So damn good. Can't believe what a mess I was until 2/4/20. The disciplined routine has freed me. I'm down in weight, down in SM/iphone screen time, up in attention to what matters, up in strength, up in spirits, up in productivity. Just up. Period. The PEERLESS system is working across the board!*

Good. Just…Good.

☞ **Give up the fleeting pleasure of eating whatever we want for the lifelong pleasure of feeling better, looking better, and living longer.**

Now that we've discussed the right food for our bodies let's discuss the right food for our minds.

CHAPTER 3

Equanimity

"The Mind is its own place:

It can make a heaven of hell or a hell of heaven."

—from *Paradise Lost,* John Milton

Do you need an old-fashioned attitude adjustment? Ask yourself this: Do you have control over your life or not? You better, or you're beaten before you begin. We make it or break it by how we take it. It starts and ends in our minds. Life is tough; we have to be tougher. Easier said than done? Not really. It's a *decision*, like everything else. A first principle. A first creation.

Being mentally tough starts by deciding to be mentally tough. As Jocko Willink so eloquently puts it: *"If you want to be tougher mentally, it is simple: Be tougher. Don't meditate on it"* (from Ferriss, *Tools*, p. 414).

Are we tough enough? Ironically, perhaps counterintuitively, being tough mentally starts with being balanced and relaxed. Composed and stable. Slowing down and taking it easy. Being equanimous. Seeking mindfulness, self-awareness, and enlightenment. And, sorry, Jocko, meditating is the very best way to get There. We can't all be Navy SEALS. But we can all be mindfully strong.

> *He who is of a calm and happy nature will hardly feel the*
> *pressure of age, but to him who is of an opposite disposition,*
> *youth and age are equally a burden.*—Plato (427-346 B.C.)

What is Equanimity?

Being calm, centered, and at peace with yourself and your surroundings. Maintaining a Buddha-like mindfulness of easy breathing, stress-free awareness, and confident acceptance of whatever *is*, knowing that *you will* prevail. You will *will* everything into existence for yourself.

> *Equanimity means not reacting to your reactions. Whatever they are. Equanimity creates a buffer around the feeling tones of experiences so that you do not react to them with craving (Hanson, Buddha's Brain, p. 117). It's a kind of shock absorber between the core of your being and whatever is passing through awareness. (Hanson, Resilient, p. 242)*

🪨 *Resilient* and *Buddha's Brain* by Rick Hanson are great resources for understanding the benefits of meditation, mindfulness, and equanimity.

> *Buddhism has a metaphor for the different conditions in life. It's called the eight worldly winds: pleasure and pain, praise and blame, gain and loss, fame and ill repute. As you develop greater equanimity, these winds have less effect on your mind. Your happiness becomes increasingly uncondi-tional, not based on catching a good breeze instead of a bad one. (Buddha's Brain, p. 117)*

When and Where Should You Strive For and Nurture Equanimity?

All the time. Morning, noon, and night. While eating, resting, writing, working out. Even playing football. Think of Tom Brady. Calm and cen-tered. In control even when he's in a rage on the sidelines. Fully aware of his surroundings, the situation, the opposing defense, his teammates, himself. Equanimity will never let you down.

Why Practice Equanimity?

Essential to all success is the state of our minds. If we're scattered, in turmoil, and out of touch with our own minds, we cannot be in touch with much else. Self-control starts with controlling our minds. We must have healthy minds firing on all eight cylinders without any malfunctioning parts. Depression, distractions, reacting rather than proacting, anxiety, and the failure to appreciate every minute of every day fully makes everything else in our lives extremely difficult to achieve. To be fully peerless, our minds must enjoy equanimity.

Chronic Stress

To reduce our stress is reason enough to strive for equanimity by practicing mindfulness and meditation. Stress kills. The studies and proof are overwhelmingly conclusive. Here's how it works: when we're stressed, our bodies release cortisol, which causes inflammation, a major contributing factor to 90% of chronic diseases. While it's true that cortisol is released when we exercise, its level returns to normal once we're done. In the case of the chronic stress we feel from everyday life—our job, our bills, our relationships, just trying to survive—those cortisol levels stay high indefinitely, thus leading to chronic inflammation. **Minimizing chronic inflammation is essential to ensuring our immune system can ward off diseases and maximize our lifespan.** So the question becomes, what can reduce stress? Nothing—I repeat, *nothing*—reduces stress as effectively and profoundly as the equanimity we achieve through mindfulness and meditation.

How Can We Test Our Stress Level?

By testing the level of C-reactive protein (CRP) in our blood since it assesses the presence of inflammation. It requires a blood draw and lab analysis, but it's well worthwhile to request the next time you have bloodwork done.

If We Suffer from Chronic Stress, What Can We Do?

As I said, seek equanimity. Look, I know there is a reluctance by many people to embrace things such as meditation, deep breathing, and other aspects of achieving equanimity because, let's face it, they tend to have connotations of softness. These eastern practices have long been perceived by some people as either unnecessary or silly. It's almost as if the average person thinks that if he or she practices deep breathing and the techniques in meditation, it's either unnecessary or a waste of time. I was one of those people. These things have been the last element of the PEERLESS system for me to embrace and believe in. Yet, everything in this peerless system could've failed for me had I not finally embraced the equanimity principles.

Regardless of what goes on around us, to us, in our lives, and in our world at large, we absolutely must maintain, nurture, and practice equanimity on a moment-to-moment basis. Keeping a calm, centered self, aids our efforts to produce, eat right, exercise, read, learn, sustain ourselves, and be successful in reaching the singularity and availing ourselves of the marvels of medical science. Everything is dependent upon equanimity.

> *The key in any kind of high-pressure situation, I think, is that 75% of success is staying calm and not losing your nerve. The rest you figure out, but once you lose your calm, everything else starts falling apart fast.* (Sam Kass, from Ferriss, *Tools*, p. 558)

The inimitable Rorke Denver, a former Navy SEAL commander, famously tells those under his command that the best piece of advice he can give them is this: *"Calm is contagious"* (from Ferriss, *Tools*, p. 91). That's genius: if we stay calm, those in our immediate circle of influence will be more likely to stay calm.

How Can We Attain and Develop a Calm Equanimity?

Again, as with everything else, it starts with the knowledge that we need to achieve it and the desire to do so.

Rick Hanson details the latest findings from neurological research that we can actually rewire our own brains. Using specific techniques, you can

> *stimulate and strengthen your brain for more fulfilling rela-*
> *tionships, a deeper spiritual life, and a greater sense of inner*
> *confidence and worth....When your mind changes, your*
> *brain changes, too....mental activity actually creates new*
> *neural structures...even fleeting thoughts can leave lasting*
> *marks on your brain.... (Buddha's Brain, back cover and*
> *p. 5)*

Noting that *"Little actions add up over time,"* Hanson suggests the following mindfulness techniques to rewire and recharge, if you will, your brain from the negative to the positive.

> *Every day, ordinary activities contain dozens of opportuni-*
> *ties to change your brain from the inside out. For example,*
> *when you are tense, take a long deep breath and let it out*
> *slowly. This activates the parasympathetic nervous system*
> *(PNS). Or when you remember an upsetting experience,*
> *immediately recall the feeling of being with someone who*
> *loves you, which will gradually infuse the upsetting memory*
> *with a positive feeling. Or to steady your mind, deliberately*
> *prolong feelings of happiness as this will increase levels of the*
> *neurotransmitter dopamine, which will help your attention*
> *and focus. (Buddha's Brain, p. 16)*

Navy SEAL Mark Divine also advocates our ability to retrain our brains, characterizing it as a 4-step process of *"starving fear and feeding courage"*:

1. *Witness negativity. Identify it and arrest it.*

2. *Interdict or stop the negative thoughts with a power statement, such as "That's negative and I despise negativity."*

3. *Redirect your mind with self-talk (such as, "I am too good, strong, and determined to allow negativity to affect me") and imagery to something positive and productive for your current goal, such as visualizing yourself having a good workout or productive session writing or closing a deal with a client.*

4. *Maintain your current state with a mantra, such as* "Every day, in every way, I'm getting better and better." (adapted from p. 28)

Ultimately, we need to discipline our thought processes because, as Jocko Willink succinctly notes, *"Discipline is freedom."*

Mindfulness

In striving for equanimity, we are disciplining our minds and conditioning our thinking by **paying attention to what we're paying attention to.** It's metathinking: **minding our own minds.**

Alas, so much of what we pay attention to throughout the day is unimportant, distracting, frustrating, negative, even worthless. Why do we pay so much attention—spend so many minutes or hours of our precious days—on stuff that does us no good whatsoever? Mainly because we're not mindful enough.

> *We're so deeply conditioned to be lost in thought and to have this conversation with ourselves from the moment we wake up to the moment we fall asleep. It's just chatter in the mind, and it's so captivating that we're not even aware of it. We are essentially in a dream state, and it's through this veil of thought that we go about our day and perceive our environment. But we are just talking to ourselves nonstop, and until you can break that spell and begin to notice thoughts themselves as objects of consciousness, just arising and passing away, you can't even pay attention to your breath, or to*

anything else, with any clarity. (Sam Harris, from Ferriss, Tools, p. 456)

Our minds wander aimlessly down mental aisles, shopping for news, gossip, and social media nonsense that is just so many shelves of other people's discards in a junk store. We dwell on negative experiences rather than tuning them out or converting them to positive ones through association techniques. We need to train ourselves to ignore 90% of it and convert the rest. *"Mindfulness is the key to regulating your attention so that you get the most out of beneficial experiences while limiting the impact of stressful, harmful ones. It enables you to recognize where your attention has gone"* (*Resilient*, p. 25-25).

Your Thoughts Are Not You

Mindfulness is all about raising our self-awareness. Who are we? What are these thoughts popping up in our minds? Throughout the day, we should always return to these fundamental questions: Who am I? Who is this thinking these thoughts? Is this thought I'm having true? If we have a disturbing or negative thought, we should return to our breath and ask ourselves: Who is this thinking? Is this thought really me? Does it serve me well to think this thought?

Realize that your thoughts are not you. They have a life of their own. If they're troubling thoughts, detach yourself from them. Question them. Where did this negative or upsetting thought come from?

If we practice this self-awareness often enough, we'll eventually automatically interrogate every dubious thought. We can't allow self-destructive, counterproductive thoughts to take over. They are not "us." One of our primary goals in life is to understand who we truly are.

As this awareness practice becomes a habit, you'll find it easier and more pleasurable to do. To state it simplistically, you'll actually begin to have fun interrogating each thought. Think of them as potential criminals, out to do you harm. Or as alien invaders, ancient bacteria, synapses gone wild. Rogue operators trying to stake a claim in the body politic which is you.

Essentially, trying to find out who you are should be one of your main concerns throughout the day. Your thoughts are trying to tell you who you are, but don't be fooled by them. Not all of them have your best interest at heart. Not all of your thoughts want you to be happy or succeed or have peace. Your thoughts very often are your own worst enemies.

At 4:30 pm on 8/3/20, while driving around doing errands, I found myself daydreaming, my mind wandering from thought to thought. I almost felt guilty and upset over having slipped out of my mental routine, my attention to mindfulness. But I reverted to the practice, started interrogating my thoughts, and asking myself who I am. My answer was and is that I'm not exactly sure, on a deep philosophical level. But on the practical and everyday level, I believe I'm the man of my Purpose, my MS, and goals. I'm the man of my focus and routine. I'm what I appear to be.

In essence, mindfulness regulates our attention so that we get the most out of beneficial experiences while limiting the impact of stressful, harmful ones. It enables us to recognize where our attention has gone. *"Being mindful means staying in the present moment as it is, moment after moment, rather than daydreaming, ruminating, or being distracted....as much research has shown, [it] lowers stress, protects health, and lifts mood"* (Resilient, p. 24).

Disclaimer: I hope that this has been clear from the first page, but it's worth stating outright that this is not a book about treating depression or pursuing *true happiness*. I'm not a doctor or a guru. If you're plagued by clinical depression, please don't think I'm proposing this system as a substitute for your doctor's treatment plan. However, whatever depression tendencies you might have and whatever lack of happiness you might feel could be at least moderately alleviated by practicing these mindfulness and meditation techniques.

For a more extensive discussion of how best to tackle depression and foster greater happiness in your life, I recommend the book *Mindfulness* by Mark Williams and Dannie Penman. They cite numerous studies indicating that regular meditation results in happier, more contented people, with a reduction in anxiety, depression, and irritability, an improvement in memory and physical stamina, a reduction in chronic stress, including hypertension, and even a reduction in chronic pain (Williams, p. 6).

That's right, research abounds supporting the contention that simply developing and practicing mindfulness can lower our stress and pain, lift our mood, and improve memory and stamina. So why would anyone *not* want to practice mindfulness?

You may doubt at this point or any point whether this is all worth it or not. It seems pretty "far out there," I know. Always asking yourself "Who am I?" may seem just a bit silly and maybe even a good deal annoying and ridiculous. "Down to earth" it's not. I get it. So you may drag your mental feet, wondering how much more of this mystical "get in touch with yourself" stuff you can handle before just wanting to return to normal, so to speak. I know. I get it. I was right there with you. But I saw so many people touting its value and effectiveness that I thought it worth further consideration. I kept my feet rooted in reality, but my mind open to the possibilities that mindfulness offers. I'm glad I did because I'm here to testify that it works. Mindfulness delivers on all its promises.

That said—with your doubts hopefully deferred if not entirely defeated— here are some action steps to move steadily forward with the program:

When in doubt, zoom out. Refocus on the big picture. Reread your MS, meditate, and repeat. (See more about dealing with doubts in Chapter 7, Sustain)

Discipline yourself to pay strict attention to your thoughts, always evaluating them for their application to your life. Put them in order, organize them, categorize them. Marshal and manage your mind.

Here's a famous SEAL mantra: *"Stay calm. Assess. Make a decision. Act."*

Here's some very practical actions you can take to assist and enhance your mindfulness:

Every time a negative thought comes up, think of someone who loves you. That rapid shifting from a negative to a positive rewires the brain so that the next time you think the same negative thought, it will instantly turn to the positive one.

- Every time you feel happy, extend that happiness as much as possible; be mindful of it. Smile. Breathe it in deeply. Make it part of you.

- Every time a dubious thought occurs to you, interrogate it by asking if it's really true. Ask yourself, "Who is this thinking this thought? Is it really me? Who am I?"

- Use your phone's "Do Not Disturb" button routinely. Do you really need instant notifications of news and texts and even phone calls? Can't they wait while you're mindful of more important things?

- Learn to "batch" activities, such as checking emails and notifications, so that you can pay better attention to your immediate tasks and concerns, rather than being constantly interrupted.

- Avoid being reactive. Don't let things that people say or things that happen during the day force an emotional reaction from you. Stay centered and calm. Be proactive.

- Make of all your words and actions an offering. Don't expect or demand anyone to respond the way you want them to. *"When you look at the things you do as offerings, they feel simpler, lighter, and more heartfelt. Even routine, seemingly trivial tasks take on new meaning and value.... We can tend to the causes but can't control the results. All we can do is make the offering"* (Resilient, pp. 232-33).

I've just scratched the surface of what Hanson has to say about mindfulness. I encourage you to read *Mindfulness, Resilience,* and *Buddha's Brain* for more insights into many other topics related to *Mindfulness* and *Equanimity.* Thich Nhat Hanh's *Peace Is Every Step* is also a charming, wise little book.

Meditation

Time to dive into the deep water. I've already prepped us a lot on land and in the pool, so to speak, so now it's time to get in the dive boat, go two miles offshore, don the scuba gear, and take the plunge. I use this metaphor because many people would not go deep water scuba diving no matter how much they were asked and encouraged to do so. Unlike deep-sea diving, Meditation is no risk at all to your health or safety. Just the opposite. Yet, I know that a significant percentage of people will balk and simply refuse to do it.

Let Me State It as Emphatically as I Can: Meditation is Essential and Priceless to Our Mental and Physical Health.

In writing *Game Changers,* Dave Asprey interviewed more than 450 of the world's most successful people from all walks of life. *"In huge numbers, they talked about meditating and using breathing techniques to find a state of peace and calm. I didn't draw that answer out of them in the interviews—it's what they actually do"* (XVI).

As part of our daily routine—being productive, eating right, exercising, reading, learning, striving for equanimity, sustaining, and working toward reversing our aging—meditating may be the glue that holds it all together. If we feel any cracks in our armor, any slippage or lizard brain torment— meditate. Feeling frustrated or angry—meditate. In pain, doubt, uncertainty—meditate. Have a chronic illness—meditate.

I used to be a skeptic, but only because I hadn't actually given it a try. What is that about people? I can't be alone in that stupid attitude of holding something in contempt that I hadn't even understood or tried, can I? Why are so many of us prone to reject out-of-hand what we know nothing about and never truly considered? Out of an inveterate lizard brain ignorance, a resistance, a fear and flight from something new. A learning-curve phobia.

Meditation Practices Living in the Present Moment

Meditation is focused attention, sometimes concentrating on a thought, mantra, or object, but often just clearing our minds entirely and focusing on our breath. Practicing how to live in the present moment. Too often, we dwell in the past or future, sacrificing our lives to what does not exist. What was is no longer, and what will be is unknown. What truly *is* is the *now*.

> *The present moment is where we have full access to our faculties. It is where we can focus on the actual task at hand and perform it masterfully. It is where our bodies are relaxed and our minds are in healthier brainwave patterns. When we learn to come back to the present moment, we have greater mental acuity.... (Shojai, pp. 33-34)*

While meditating, we're openly monitoring and observing our breath, and training our brains to live in the present.

> *I almost feel like by not meditating before, my brain was sitting on the couch.* (Adam Fisher, from Ferriss, Tools, p. 430)

Don't let your brain be a couch-potato. Among all self-help practices, meditation reigns supreme:

> *It is a meta-skill that improves everything else. You're starting your day by practicing focus when it doesn't matter (sitting on a couch for 10 minutes) so that you can focus better later when it does matter (negotiation, conversation with a loved one, max deadlift, mind-melding with a Vulcan, etc.).* (Ferriss, Tools, p. 149)

The unbridled praise for meditation is universal and convincing:

> *...Meditation [is] a way to relinquish control of my conscious mind so that my more powerful unconscious mind [can] take over, and my analysis of the world [can] improve.... Meditation is one of the most practical, powerful, productivity-enhancing tools ever created, and learning to meditate is one of the best investments I ever made. (Adam Robinson, from Ferriss, Tribe, p. 189)*

How Should We Meditate?

There are literally thousands of elaborate meditations described at exhausting length in hundreds of books and websites.

If you want a definitive book on meditation, read *Mindfulness* by Mark Williams and Danny Penman. Jam-packed with dozens of different types of meditations, it's a highly detailed guide, including a step-by-step eight-week plan. It's great.

If you want to experience the high-priced, boutique form of meditation, be like David Lynch: "*Learn Transcendental Meditation as taught by Maharishi Mahesh Yogi and meditate regularly. This will end your suffering and give you happiness and fulfillment in life. Rock on!*" (David Lynch, from Ferriss,

Tools, p. 379) Maharishi famously taught the Beatles, among others, about Transcendental Meditation. Lynch has a website and course to teach you: https://www.davidlynchfoundation.org/.

India's Vedic tradition of Transcendental Consciousness (TC) was studied by Ralph Waldo Emerson, who introduced it to Henry David Thoreau, who put it into practice by living for two years in a cabin in the woods he immortalized in his classic, *Walden*. While there, he reached TC's *fourth major state of consciousness:* beyond waking, dreaming, and sleeping, where your mind transcends mere thoughts and feelings.

> *If with closed ears and eyes I consult consciousness for a moment, immediately are all walls and barriers dissipated, earth rolls from under me, and I float....No sun illumines me, for I dissolve all lesser lights in my own intenser and steadier light....To be calm, to be serene! There is the calmness of the lake when there is not a breath of wind....So it is with us. Sometimes we are clarified and calmed healthily, as we never were before in our lives, not by an opiate, but by some unconscious obedience to the all-just laws, so that we become like a still lake of purest crystal and without an effort our depths are revealed to ourselves. All the world goes by us and is reflected in our deeps. Such clarity!—Thoreau's Journals*

It's going to take some time before I make it *There*, to Thoreau's level, but I can try.

First things first. One step at a time.

Your First Step is Learning to Breathe

All meditation, indeed all relaxation, calmness, refocusing, reenergizing, and recovery begins and ends with breathing.

The breath carries our life force. It is our connection with the essential nature of the Universe and our anchor into the Great Mystery itself. The expansion and contraction of the very Universe is mirrored in our breath. (Shojai, p. 15)

<u>Conscious breathing</u>. You can't find a single article, book, website, or video about meditating that doesn't focus on breathing. During my entire life, going way back to my teenage years, somewhere, in something I read, I learned about the importance of drinking water and taking deep breaths. On hundreds of occasions, I've delighted in annoying people—friends, family, foes—by this comeback to their comments, anger, frustration in arguments, or even conflicts with me by smiling and saying, "Take a deep breath." I always mean it, but it's often taken as a wiseass passive/aggressive attack on them. I don't know why. Taking a deep breath—preferably 3 or 4, slowly, holding it in, and exhaling, counting to 3 on each action—almost always has a calming, focusing effect.

Almost all meditations, as I said, revolve around clearing your mind by focusing on your breath, your breathing. Becoming aware of only your breath, of only the act of breathing in and breathing out. When a thought occurs, let it go, returning to the breath. In your daily meditating, you are taking 10-15 minutes to practice strengthening your control over your own thoughts—thoughts that are not you and are often harmful to your best interest. Practice focusing on your breathing, and you'll eventually be using a 30-second version of this technique any and every time throughout the day that you feel stressed or upset. Just take 30 seconds to return to your breath, letting go of your thoughts, and clearing your mind. This 30-second practice will soon become your go-to method of regaining your composure and strength. There's really nothing as powerful to help you regain and maintain like conscious breathing.

The wonderful, wise meditation teacher Thich Nhat Hanh speaks rhapsodically about breathing:

Breathing in and out is very important and it is enjoyable. Our breathing is the link between our body and our mind. Sometimes our mind is thinking of one thing and our body is doing another, and mind and body are not unified. By concentrating on our breathing, "In" and "Out," we bring body and mind back together, and become whole again. Conscious breathing is an important bridge. (Hanh, p. 9)

Many meditation sessions described in books and guided in videos and podcasts begin by telling us to close our eyes and start our conscious breathing by visualizing our breath going in and out of our lungs. We are told to bring our attention to our chests and picture our lungs taking our breath in and out.

Because I believe in visual learning, I thought it would help see actual lungs in operation. It was. Now, when I close my eyes and practice breathing, I know much better what the lungs and diaphragm look like and what they're doing as my chest inflates and deflates.

Here are a few links to good videos about what the lungs look like, how they work, and what they do:

How do we breathe? The lungs and diaphragm work together to bring oxygen into the lungs and to move carbon dioxide out of your lungs. The diaphragm is a large muscle that is found under your lungs. Your lungs are actually composed of millions of tiny air sacs and depend on the diaphragm in order to inflate. https://tinyurl.com/y3dv4lua *(MooMooMath and Science, 10/24/18)*

This one is by Florida Hospital Kissimmee Lung Anatomy Animation. Its context is a doctor explaining the lung's functions to patients with lung cancer. https://youtu.be/ibqFS7wusG4 *(4/9/12) https://tinyurl.com/y6czwc3t* (*"How healthy lungs work and function", 9/22/13, by 3D Mania*)

Once Again: Learn to Tame Your Thoughts

Meditation has many purposes—to relieve stress, take a time out from your day, calm down, "get in touch with your feelings" etc.—but perhaps its fundamental objective and benefit is to master your own thoughts. As we've said, your thoughts are not you. They're products of millions of synaptic impulses, random firings of neurons, rogue imposters, traitors, and other assorted invading voices that do not define us. Don't identify with all your thoughts. Be wary of them. Learn to note them with a disinterested curiosity. They can zip and bounce and scurry around in your head, all competing for your attention, but don't attach yourself to them.

Tamara Levitt insightfully explains this practice of noting your thoughts without identifying with them in her "Staying Afloat" practice:

> *If there are any thoughts or emotions, notice them without identifying with them, without getting sucked into them. We want to feel what's happening in the present moment without referring to a me or a self. So you can notice thinking, but it's not you in the thinking. Thinking is simply happening. So just say "thinking, thinking." And notice emotions. Perhaps there's anger. But it's not you in the anger. There's simply the experience of anger so just observe it and say "anger, anger." And say it over and over until you can feel the anger without it becoming you. And then gently come back to your body, feeling the rise of your breath as it enters your lungs.*

Tamara shares a couple of tools to shield us from anger, and I would add nastiness, hostility, unkindness, aggression, and other toxic responses directed at us:

...such as imagining a protective space around us so that when anger is propelled toward you, you can imagine it bouncing off this protective layer. That way, aggression is deflected and has a place to land. We can also try noting the emotions of others just as we note our own emotions. Noting helps create distance between us and our experience, almost as if we are watching a film. When we observe emotions in this way, we can cushion their impact and avoid reacting to them. So if someone is being critical, we can note criticism. If they are angry, we can note anger. When we step back and observe anger as a spectator, it feels less personal and less hurtful. As the saying goes, ships don't sink because of the water around them; they sink because of the water that gets into them. So when anger is directed toward you, reach for these tools and create some distance from what's happening, protect yourself, and stay afloat. (Calm App, 11/05/20)

My Specific Meditations

I like simple myself. "*Simplify! Simplify!*" Thoreau shouted at us. I got the message. Keeping it simple is particularly practical when getting started. We can always build on our knowledge and add to our bag of tricks later on. Too much information can be confusing and discouraging, especially when we have many other projects and goals to focus on (such as producing, eating right, exercising, reading, learning, work, family, etc.).

So here's a very simple meditation to get us started: Allocate 10 minutes for yourself. Find a quiet place. Sit erect in a chair, your spine straight and your hands comfortable in your lap. Focus on clearing your mind and practicing thought management. Close your eyes and take a few deep breaths. 4 seconds in. 2 seconds hold. 4 seconds out. Observe your lungs. Call upon the videos to picture your lungs in detail. Really see your own lungs in your chest while you're breathing. If other thoughts intrude, recognize them give them space, observe them, but don't identify with them. And slowly dismiss them, letting them float off like clouds in the sky. Your mind is a blue sky, your thoughts random clouds floating by. Return to your breathing. Focus, breathe, repeat. Try to go deeper, feeling yourself tuning out everything around you.

That's it. Simple as that.

That's a go-to meditation for me. I've also developed another, alternative meditation as of 8/16/20. It's very stream-of-consciousness gratitude practice, allowing for thoughts to take their own course, guided by appreciation and joy

I go out on my pool patio in the morning. While I do various back and torso stretches, I launch into a stream-of-consciousness gratefulness celebration of my life, my house, my pool, my backyard, all the colors of the trees and bushes and plants, the blue sky, the blue water, the spa waterfall and the two fountains into the pool, the splashing, soothing sound of the water, the light reflecting off it, how I am "imbibing good health opening my mouth to the wind" (Thoreau), the very fact that this oasis is mine, my personal peaceful oasis. I stretch and breathe and enjoy the sights and sounds...all 5 senses engaged. So grateful this is mine, and my youngest son and wife are asleep inside, and grown daughters and older son are safe and secure in their houses and all of them love me. I am loved. I revisit my MS, grateful for its solidity, and my Goals, both short and long term. I am so grateful for my routine, for being organized, structured, disciplined. I go through the letters in my *PEERLESS* system...immensely grateful for having cobbled and hammered it into shape. So grateful for all of life's opportunities and for this beautiful day and extraordinary environment I've been blessed with....I am blessed and I am breathing deeply and taking in all the pool slashing sounds and the trees and colors and the two birds flying overhead....just everything natural and manmade in harmony here in my oasis. I compose my own Whitmanesque "Song of Myself" ... I am large, I contain multitudes...I am 70, but getting younger, stronger, better every day...I will not waver, I will face all obstacles and setbacks by saying "good"... I like the obstacles and setbacks, they will prove that I am strong for I will overcome them and stay the course, not just surviving but thriving, for I have my MS, my gratitude, my daily, weekly, monthly, yearly goals and action plans and principles of fortitude and strength of mind and self-discipline to soldier on…

That's something like how it goes. Very stream-of-consciousness. For me, it's not about reaching a deep, thoughtless meditative state in the morning. For me—and you can do this in any way you want, obviously—the morning meditation wakes me up, makes me grateful and happy, and energizes me to get started writing and then the gym and then tackling all the business and personal chores and challenges.

Get to "*There*": Your Life and the Lives of Your Loved Ones May Depend on It

In the morning, I'm just trying to get to a place where I can get to work. I may be wrong, and I'm sure some meditation gurus will dismiss my methods and advice as wrongheaded, but they work for me. *Later* in the day, *after* I get my work done, I meditate the "*right*" way, the *deep* way, the way that leads me to "*There.*"

I haven't heard any experts, practitioners, or teachers of meditation that I've read or quoted so far—though admittedly, I've barely scratched the surface in the meditation world—talk about *There.*

William Butler Yeats—whose first volume of poetry, "*The Wind Among the Reeds,*" published in 1899, ushered in the Modern era in poetry—was always seeking what he called "*There,*" with a capital T. "*There*" is some center, some ultimate spiritual reality that made sense, that held everything together. He was quite the transcendent, meditative mystic. Always exploring occult traditions; always seeking some unified explanation of the world and the soul.

The forces of chaos and fear in the world are standing in the way of our finding *There.* How is one to reach an inner meditative state of peace, mindfulness, serenity, and calm with such horrific and potentially catastrophic events happening in our country and world? Yet, the question should actually be: How can we *not* seek the soothing centering refuge that mindful meditation and our own personal *There* offer us? We could safely argue that in the 2020's, more than ever before, we desperately *need* to be peerless, focused, attentive, mindful, transcendent, and *There*, for ourselves and our families.

Yeats knew how imperative it was to have control of yourself in a world spinning out of control.

In his most famous poem, "The Second Coming"—one of the five best poems in the English language—Yeats prophesied the coming horror of the 20th century. Without knowing exactly what was to come, his *"rough beast slouching toward Bethlehem to be born,"* came true in the personages of Lenin, Mao, Hitler, Stalin, Mussolini, Pol-Pot, Amin, Castro, Hussein, and the other mass-murdering totalitarian dictators of the past 100 years.

Turning and turning in the widening gyre

The falcon cannot hear the falconer;

Things fall apart; the centre cannot hold;

Mere anarchy is loosed upon the world,

The blood-dimmed tide is loosed, and everywhere

The ceremony of innocence is drowned;

The best lack all conviction, while the worst

Are full of passionate intensity.

Surely some revelation is at hand;

Surely the Second Coming is at hand.

The Second Coming! Hardly are those words out

When a vast image out of Spiritus Mundi

Troubles my sight: somewhere in sands of the desert

A shape with lion body and the head of a man,

A gaze blank and pitiless as the sun,

Is moving its slow thighs, while all about it

Reel shadows of the indignant desert birds.

The darkness drops again; but now I know

That twenty centuries of stony sleep

Were vexed to nightmare by a rocking cradle,

And what rough beast, its hour come round at last,

Slouches towards Bethlehem to be born?

"*Things fall apart; the centre cannot hold...The blood-dimmed tide is loosed... innocence is drowned....the worst are filled with passionate intensity....*"

Sound at all familiar nowadays?

If you care to know more, read my short article about Yeats: *http://www. drmarcdbaldwin.com/2011/09/5-exceedingly-deep-writing-tips-from-william-butler-yeats/*. It's a chapter from my book *Writing Fabulous Fiction*: (https://edit911.com/pdfs/Writing_Fabulous_Fiction.pdf).

Gratitude

Quite a segue: from things falling apart and the impending doomsday of the 2020s, to being grateful! But again, in **gratitude is refuge from the storm.**

A big part of everything meaningful in life is our *need* to be grateful. Feeling blessed. Counting your blessings. My morning stream-of-consciousness meditation—and refocusing all day long—centers around gratitude.

> *I don't just think gratitude. I let gratitude fill my soul, because when you're grateful, we all know there's no anger. It's impossible to be angry and grateful simultaneously. When you're grateful, there is no fear. You can't be fearful and grateful simultaneously. (Robbins, from Ferriss, Tools, p. 214)*

🌾 We can actively practice gratitude by thinking of at least three things that we're grateful for. Think of those three things and then totally focus on feeling the presence of God. If you're not a believer in God, focus on whatever larger force or meaning in life that you do believe in. Fate? The Force? The Universe? The Big Bang? Nothingness? Existentialism? Focus on those. And then expand your focus into *wanting* and *envisioning*. Focus on what you *want to happen* for yourself, your goals, your life, your loved ones, today, tomorrow...and then *visualize* those goals and desires *actually happening, actually coming true.*

I could travel all around the world, read all the books on meditation, and I'm sure I'd conclude, as I did this morning, that what I'm most grateful for and the best place for me is in my own backyard. Home.

"We must cultivate our garden" – *Candide*

After my 10-15 minutes cultivating myself on the patio by my pool, I'm so happy I can't wait to get to work. It's wondrous how wonderful it makes me feel.

Gratitude is also good for your heart. *"Positive feelings such as appreciation create increased order and balance in the autonomic nervous system, resulting in enhanced immunity, improved hormonal balance, and more efficient brain function"* (Childre, p. 46).

Heart Rate Variability (HRV)

Speaking of your heart, yet another reason to meditate is that it *is*, in fact, good for your heart because it decreases stress as it regulates your heartbeat. An increasingly more popular approach to meditating is to do so in conjunction with measuring your pulse and heart rate.

> *HRV measures the spacing between each heartbeat and compares it to the spacing of other individual heartbeats. When you are in a state of fight or flight, your HRV becomes*

very flat, with equal spacing between heartbeats but when you are in a restful state of flow, the variability of your heart rate may go up or down, but the HRV increases dramatically. The spacing between two heartbeats will be much different from the spacing between two other heartbeats that come a moment later. Your HRV impacts everything from your brain waves to your cardiovascular health and even the people around you. (Asprey, Game Changers, p. 260).

Doc Childre, the founder of HeartMath Institute and author of *The Heartmath Solution*, explains the importance of HRV this way: "*Our emotional states are reflected in our heart rhythms, as seen in heart rate variability measurements. Our heart rhythms affect the brain's ability to process information, make decisions, solve problems, and experience and express creativity*" (Childre, p. 46). Thus, when we meditate and breathe consciously, such focusing on our heart, "*improves nervous system balance, heightens cardiovascular efficiency, and enhances communication between heart and brain, bringing more coherence to the mind and emotions*" (Childre, p. 69).

HRV Training Apps

Several different companies offer HRV training, with apps for teaching and monitoring, and sensors for registering various readings. I checked two of them, buying their $165 sensors, and downloading and using their apps.

<u>Inner Balance</u>

The sensor clips onto your ear lobe. It's not uncomfortable. It syncs via Bluetooth with the app. However, sorry to report that I used it four times to monitor my HRV and all four times I had difficulty getting it to sync. It sent me on a loop of not recognizing or finding the sensor 2, 3, even 4 times. Finally, I got it to sync. There's a simplistic color wheel you stare at to get your breathing in sync with their preferred rhythm. It's somewhat unpleasant staring at it, truthfully. The readings, though better than nothing, aren't anything special. The extras—resources, training, other programs—aren't much to get excited about either, frankly.

Yet, I'm not comfortable giving it a negative review. If there were no other HRV apps, sensors, and training available, IB would be fine. But there is, and their competition is better.

<u>Elite HRV by Heartmath Solutions</u>

Developed by the HeartMath Institute, Elite HRV has its CoreSense monitor, a fingertip design, much like a doctor's office uses to measure the pulse. Much more comfortable than the IB one. And their App also provides far superior feedback, more complete and insightful. Their system, book, and app are the real deal. I use it every day, and its accuracy is uncanny and even unnerving. When I just don't feel right in the morning, the app's readings corroborate my poor state, telling me I'm not in good shape to exercise much. When I feel great in the morning, the readings also tell me I feel great. By recording daily readings, I'm setting a biomarker graph for myself that I can use as one more tool to track my health.

Get a Meditation Phone App Such as *Calm*

I highly recommend getting an app for your phone and using 10-12 minute guided meditations, at least to get you started. I checked out a dozen different apps, and my favorite is Calm. Again, I have no vested interest in or connection to Calm. I'm recommending it because it's great. Their lead instructor is Tamara Levitt. I cannot speak highly enough about how good she is at what she does. A true professional. It's pure pleasure to be a student of hers. I enjoy her meditations so much, I do 2 or 3 of them every day. She wrote and narrates perhaps 300 or more meditations on many different topics, and they're all effective, insightful, and often brilliant. I've listened to some of them 3 or 4 times, they're that good.

What if We're Having Trouble Focusing During Meditation?

It can be very hard to keep our minds clear when meditating. Our minds wander. Maybe our to-do list, or disturbing or troubling thoughts of various problems, make it hard to focus and pay attention to our meditating.

If that happens, Tamara Leavitt recommends this technique:

> *Try allowing for whatever comes up without resistance. Bring an openness to your practice by silently reciting the phrase: "May I meet this moment fully. May I meet it as a friend." When we open to the moment with friendliness, we can shift the way in which we experience it. "May I meet this moment fully. May I meet it as a friend." This is how we can meet each thought, each emotion, each breath. ("Gorillas," Daily Calm)*

In this way, we turn the negative into positive, disarming the negative by approaching it proactively rather than reactively.

☙ So, have you tried meditation yet? If not, try it now. Use either the first one or a modification of my own. It doesn't have to be formal or elaborate. You're just getting started. You can develop and improve your meditation practice as the days and weeks go by. Here's a good video to check out: https://www.youtube.com/watch?v=iN6g2mr0p3Q.

☙ Trust me and download the *Calm* app. Buy a monthly subscription and let Tamara be your guide. She's really good!

☠ You may ask again, why? What's the point of meditating? I still don't get it or need it. The simple and profound answer is that meditating *will* improve your life. *"More than 80% of the world-class performers I've interviewed have some form of daily meditation or mindfulness practice"* (Ferriss, *Tools*, p. 149).

Review of Some Specific Aspects of Meditating

- Repeat these mantras and come up with some of your own:

  - Every day, in every way, I'm getting better and better.

  - I am a construction project. I am better with structure. I am con-structing myself: building myself with this structure.

  - Only the strong survive.

  - The purpose of life is a life of purpose.

  - I will work on me with a sense of urgency. I cannot wait for me to get better and better.

  - Good.

  - Grin and bear it.

  - Only the strong survive.

  - Do me.

  - Diet, Gym, Work, Read.

  - Pay attention to what you're paying attention to. Pay attention only to your circle of influence; ignore the circle of concern.

- Mentally skim over PEERLESS, slowing down and dwelling on key elements relevant to the specific moment, situation, or difficulty you're facing.

- Talk positively to yourself: "*I'm strong, I'm capable, I can deal with this, I can do this. Nothing is beyond my ability to handle.*"

- Recall your MS & Goals.

- Practice conscious breathing.

- Practice gratitude.

Just now (8/18/20 @7:28 am), as I grabbed a book to add notes right here about meditating on gratefulness, I stopped and caught myself being productive and grateful, and grateful for my productivity. The thought gave me chills. That's how I know I'm getting it. I'm learning, growing, getting mentally stronger. *"I'm following my plan to write by opening this book to find a quote to add right here. I'm so grateful to be alive, awake, paying attention, using my brain, writing. HEAL. I am having this experience. Enriching it by skimming over all the elements of mindfulness, absorbing the experience of positively reinforcing myself with self-talk and gratitude, just celebrating how far I've come in the past 6 months, 6 weeks, even 6 days. Everything is falling into place. Everything relates. My synapses of the system are firing together and wiring together. Synchronicity is occurring."*

The Power of Gone

An ordained Shingon monk, Shinzen Young, who now teaches meditation in the U.S., espouses his *"Just Note Gone"* as *the* most important focus technique of all.

We spend so much time noting the start and duration of a sensation or feeling, but not when it's gone. For example, we get insulted by a rude remark or angry sitting in a traffic jam or freshly tormented by a troubling memory or worried over a piece of bad news. We experience mental and emotional pain at the onset of those negative feelings, and throughout the duration of our paying attention to them. They bother us until they depart our minds, and our attention turns to other thoughts. But we rarely say good riddance to them. We never thoroughly wash our hands of them or absolve ourselves of their negative effect.

Young explains how and why we should "just note gone" when a sensation or thought suddenly disappears from our mind:

> *Clearly acknowledge when you detect the transition point between all of it being present and at least some of it no*

longer being present. Why should we care about whether we can detect the moment when a particular burst of mental talk or a particular external sound or a particular body sensation suddenly subsides?... Under such extreme duress, is there anywhere you can turn to find relief? Yes. You can concentrate intently on the fact that each sensory insult passes. In other words, you can reverse the normal habit of turning to each new arising and instead turn to each new passing. **Micro-relief is constantly available.**

With time, the "Just Note Gone" technique will sensitize you to detect vanishings more clearly. This combined with the equanimity loop makes it possible to concentrate continuously on vanishings. This in turn transforms micro-ending into mega-relief. Noting "gone" produces other positive effects in addition to a sense of relief. Some people find that noticing moments of vanishing creates a deep sense of restfulness. Visual, auditory, or somatic tranquility may seem to propagate through consciousness whenever you notice a "gone." Each moment of cessation points to absolute rest— the still point of the turning world.

Calmness and peace reside in that "still point of the turning world." In that zone, we find mindfulness.

Transcendentalism

At this point, it's worth developing the growing realization I'm having—on 8/20/20 @ 7:14 am—that reaching a calm meditative state equates with **finding your inner self by transcending this external, outside world.** Right now, as I'm writing and thinking about it, I'm getting more peaceful and detached from all distractions and the unimportant things in life. Transcendentalism teaches that reality is spiritual or ideal rather than material. Perhaps the primary intention and objective of meditation— breathing deeply, working on calming our minds—is to reach a transcendent state, a place where we *"get in touch with our true feelings and nature."*

I know. It can all sound cliched and like hippy-dippy nonsense. But that impression comes from a place of doubt and rigidity, from the mind having been made up and closed down. I've been there. But I've also been schooled in—and taught to thousands of my students—the history and literature of transcendentalism, from Hindu texts to Ralph Waldo Emerson and Henry David Thoreau. Transcendentalism, mindfulness, and meditation comprise one interconnected body of thought that teaches the importance and joy of developing *our selves* by tuning out the distractions and white noise of the world.

Self-Reliance

In his must-read classic, *Self-Reliance,* Emerson urges us to transcend our reliance upon the concerns and things of this world to find fulfillment within our selves: *"Nothing can bring you peace but yourself. Nothing can bring you peace but the triumph of principles."* The quest for that "triumph" begins by codifying our principles in our MS. *Self-Reliance* is Emerson's MS, wherein he details the principles of freedom rooted in discipline.

Through our self-reliance, we can reach the *Over-Soul,* an inner light or animating force, where the *"me"* and the *"not me"* are joined. All of nature is *"not me"* while only the *Over-Soul* is *"me."* This concept is the equivalent of William Wordsworth's *"spots of time"* in which we transcend this world and become one with nature. When we are meditating, it is a *"spot of time"* where we attempt to join the *"not me"* and the *"me."*

So, what's the relevance of all this 19th-century spiritualism? For me, just embracing nature and the sense that there's a much bigger universe of which I'm a part is comforting. It's at once humbling and motivating. When we "get it," we tap into the *Spiritus Mundi,* the collective unconscious of the world, allowing us to make connections with the same thoughts and brainwaves that have flowed through billions of minds before ours.

Childlike Sense of Wonder

Yes, it's all very much "far out there," perhaps. But the Eastern traditions—namely Buddhism and Hinduism—are famous for having produced peaceful, calm, happy people. We don't have to chuck our whole lives, become monks, wear robes, and live cross-legged in temples chanting mantras all day. Not a lot of Buddhists do that anyway. What we can do that's extremely beneficial to us is just pay attention, be mindful, and appreciate and be grateful for all the wondrous things in life.

Thoreau—just to stick with one human being who sought his inner self and connection with nature and the collective unconscious—looked at the world with innocence, *"striving to recover the lost child that I am....It is only when we forget all our learning that we begin to know....[because] the highest wisdom does not inspect, but behold."*

This frame of mind is also perfectly illustrated by Walt Whitman in his superb poem *"When I Heard the Learn'd Astronomer"*:

When I heard the learn'd astronomer,
When the proofs, the figures, were ranged in columns before me,
When I was shown the charts and diagrams, to add, divide, and measure them,
When I sitting heard the astronomer where he lectured with much applause in the lecture-room,
How soon unaccountable I became tired and sick,
Till rising and gliding out I wander'd off by myself,
In the mystical moist night-air, and from time to time,
Look'd up in perfect silence at the stars.

The grand irony is that the more we seek ourselves and our individuality, the more we come to believe in the collective unconscious of humanity . As Thoreau said, *"If I seem to boast more than is becoming, my excuse is that I brag for humanity rather than for myself."* This statement echoes many of Walt Whitman's lines—such as *"I am large, I contain multitudes"* and *"If you want me again, look for me under your bootsoles."*

We are not alone. That's the key. **There's an infinitely vast *spirit of the world* and a *not-me* and an *Over-Soul* and *Nature* and a *collective unconscious* out *There* that we can tap in to if only we try.**

Intuition

We all have inside us an innate ability to acquire knowledge unconsciously, by our inner selves. Emerson uses his "intuition" to "see truly." Nirvana is the ultimate goal: a deep state of inner peace. Wouldn't that be nice? We can doubt it, scoff at it, or truly consider it. Does such a state of Nirvana actually exist? If so, I want to go *There*. Who *wouldn't* want deep inner peace?

The Ultimate Goal of All Eastern Spirituality: Wisdom

All of these mind games—seeking equanimity, calm, our *Over-Soul, Spiritus Mundi, There,* and Nirvana through mindful meditation—have as one of their ultimate goals the **quest for wisdom.**

Wisdom means that we can identify and understand Truth and Beauty. What is inherently and universally and infinitely true and good. Not the fads, the fleeting, the momentary. The timeless.

Such absolute standards are scoffed and condemned in this radically relativistic world today. But there *are* some absolutes, some unchanging truths. Inside us all, we can find our Truth and Beauty if we clear our minds of the cobwebs and smokescreens.

In another of the five greatest Romantic poems ever written, *"Ode on a Grecian Urn,"* John Keats expresses our search for the undying, eternal standards. We all want a mooring in the cosmic dock, a place we can call home, the knowledge and wisdom of unchanging principles and beliefs that transcend believing and reach unshakeable fact.

> *When old age shall this generation waste,*
>
> *Thou shalt remain, in midst of other woe*
>
> *Than ours, a friend to man, to whom thou say'st,*
>
> *"Beauty is truth, truth beauty—that is all*
>
> *Ye know on earth, and all ye need to know."*

Truth is beautiful and what's beautiful is true.

But in our material world, made ever more complicated by relativity, the questions and the seeking of answers remain: How do we define truth and beauty? The answer: Inside our intuitive minds, alive with a sense of wonder about the natural world around and within us.

Yet, we've all been misled, steered off a better course for our lives, by the outside world. Most of us are *not* mindful of what's truly important. We've shut down. Our eyes do not see, our ears do not hear. We rush around with little connection to *our selves*, accepting what's false and ugly, settling for mediocrity.

In *"The World Is Too Much With Us"*—yet another of the five greatest Romantic poems ever written, and one of the penultimate transcendentalist poems of the Romantic Period (the teenage years of Transcendentalism)— Wordsworth decries this "wast[ing]" of our lives:

The world is too much with us; late and soon

> *Getting and spending, we lay waste our powers;*

Little we see in Nature that is ours;

We have given our hearts away, a sordid boon!

This Sea that bares her bosom to the moon;

The winds that will be howling at all hours,

And are up-gathered now like sleeping flowers;

For this, for everything, we are out of tune;

It moves us not. Great God! I'd rather be

A Pagan suckled in a creed outworn;

So might I, standing on this pleasant lea,

Have glimpses that would make me less forlorn;

Have sight of Proteus rising from the sea;

Or hear old Triton blow his wreathèd horn.

What a poem! I always loved reading it aloud to my students and teaching them about its genius, its Truth and Beauty.

As a relevant aside to our project of becoming peerless, notice that it's a sonnet. A sonnet is a very distinct way of structuring a poem. It's 14 lines of iambic pentameter—10 syllables in 5 beats a line. "*The world. Is too. Much with. Us late. And soon.*" Of course, we don't *read* it like that. We read it naturally. But the underlying structure of the lines gives it its power. The seeming rigidity of the form, paradoxically, gives it its mellifluous rhythm.

"*Discipline is freedom.*" In both life and poetry, **strength comes from structure, from the system.**

Notice, also, its interesting end rhyme scheme. 4 quatrains and an ending couplet. Enjoy how the first line rhymes with the fourth, and the second line rhymes with the third, and so on: abba, abba, cdcd, cd.

Such form. Such discipline. Such freedom accorded by the system. Such Truth. Such Beauty.

For a fuller discussion of Transcendentalism, watch my lecture: https://www.youtube.com/watch?v=UJx_q5bILCE&t=11s.

Paying Attention Like a Transcendentalist

<u>What it boils down to is this: we need to pay much better and closer attention to the natural world around and inside us</u>. We need to actively look for and enhance transcendent, insightful (*in-sight-ful*: what we see *inside*, seeing the *inside of* things and thoughts) experiences, **paying attention** to them for as long as possible. In this way, **we are rewiring our brains.** *"The longer something is held in awareness the more neurons fire and wire together and the stronger the trace in memory"* (Hanson, *Buddha's Brain,* pp. 68-9).

Our attitudes and moods are profoundly affected by everything in our lives. So we need to **pay attention to what we're paying attention to.** *We must "manage our attention. Who we become, what we learn and accomplish, and who's with us in the end will ensue directly from the things we pay the most attention to day after day and year after year"* (Matthews, p. 67).

Don't lose your focus on what's most important in your life: the elements in your MS, your Goals, your daily schedule, your family, yourself. When a distracting or negative thought such as a bad experience comes to mind, immediately think of a positive experience or a positive outcome. In that way, the negative thoughts and experiences become wired to and automatically associated with the positive experience. *"Over time, the accumulating impact of this positive material will literally, synapse by synapse, change your brain"* (Hanson, *Buddha's Brain,* p. 71). Keep re-minding yourself of optimistic, upbeat, positive memories.

Constantly Refocus

"The single thing that most prevents success... Is always focus [or lack of focus]. I believe focus is the key to everything. So, figuring out how to find

focus or get back to my focus is something I ponder a lot" (**Tim McGraw, from Ferriss,** *Tools***, p. 465**).

Paying attention and focusing mirror and complement proactivity and extreme ownership, taking personal responsibility for everything in our lives, including our thoughts. Recognizing that it's all up to us. *"The proactive approach is to change from the inside-out: to be different and by being different, to affect positive change in what's out there—I can be more resourceful, I can be more diligent, I can be more creative, I can be more cooperative"* (Covey, p. 89).

Another strategy is to treat our quest for equanimity and focus like a sport: there's practice and then there are games. If we practice well, we're more likely to play well. During practice (reading, researching, thinking), we continually learn more about rewiring, meditation, and mindfulness techniques, setting aside specific practice times to do so. During the "games" (our everyday activities, work, socializing, living life), we can then shift into short meditations and mindfulness techniques. We can remind ourselves to refocus, pay attention, be proactive. We can call upon those techniques anytime and anywhere, in any situation where we need to gain, maintain, or restore control, calm, and order within ourselves and/or our surroundings.

When Serious, Real Problems Foil Our Attempts to "Meditate Them Away"

I'm fully aware that it's all well and good to say "just meditate, do some conscious breathing, refocus, be happy, be grateful" when we're tired, troubled, worried, or stressed. But life throws real and serious problems at us that meditation and mindfulness won't solve. When we have very real worries, concerns, or issues that are pressing and painful, what specifically can we do at the moment? When closing our eyes and doing conscious breathing won't cure what ails us, what do we do?

Let's acknowledge and recognize that mindful meditation was never meant to be a cure. It's meant to help us calm our minds so we're better positioned mentally to *find* the cures and solutions for problems—or at least the next steps to take to address them proactively.

So, after we've meditated, what do we do next to address the serious issues that don't just magically evaporate because we're in a mindful state of mind?

What *do* we do when we think our spouse is cheating on us? Or our son is taking drugs? Or our job is getting worse all the time and we're either going to be fired or have to quit? Or we've had a terrifying health diagnosis and we may have cancer?

Meditate. That's right: slow it down, try to calm down, and then...

Then, get to work. Work the system. Be productive, write, read, learn, sustain our efforts.

I'd start by opening a Gdoc and writing.

Write down the specific issue or problem. Be as clear and detailed about it as you can. What's the worst-case scenario and the best-case scenario?

- Brainstorm possible proactive approaches and solutions. What are as many courses of action that we can think of taking?

- Research Google. See what other people have done about this problem. See what the "experts" suggest. Just type in the specific issue. I just typed in "what do I do if I think my kid is taking drugs" and 193 million entries came up. Usually, the best ones are on the first few pages. Lots of articles by doctors, psychologists, counselors, and addiction specialists. Read through them, take notes, and add the possible actions to our Gdoc.

- From there, narrow down the choices and write our Goals for this problem and potential Action Plans. What steps can we take today, this week, this month, and permanently to address this problem?

- Now we have things down in writing. We have resources to advise us.

- Try to keep a cool head—meditate some more—look over our Gdoc and make a decision. What's our best course of action?

When facing a serious problem, we might let ourselves get derailed. Some problems are so big, most people would understand if we temporarily "lost it."

I don't want to sound insensitive, but our MS and Goals to become peerless simply can't be put aside. No matter what, we *must* press on. In fact, we need our system and routine more than ever. It will help us cope, keep cool, and figure out what to do next, the rest of today, tomorrow, and on into the future. Fall back on it. Rely on it. The system is the solution.

Supplemental Es

As always, these letters instantly recall key words that trigger a chain of thoughts to run through our minds quickly. Just as I'm recapitulating and reminding us why we're encoding our system in words with the same first letter, we need to constantly repeat everything to ourselves, hardwiring our brains, getting our synapses to fire automatically in positive paths.

By *Energizing* ourselves many times a day through repeating our mantras and positive self-talk, we're rewiring our brains. Gradually, but eventually and definitely, our responses to external or internal negative stimuli will be automatic. In other words, this entire system will become systematic. Everything gets easier and more efficient the more we do it. Practice makes perfect. Positive energy feeds itself.

Feel *Excited* by our goals over *Embracing* the system. I get excited about what I'm doing, about life itself. I visualize myself succeeding. By this *Envisioning* of my daily routine, I get pumped up and *Excited.* If we can be excited about life, then we're alive.

If we've given a great *Effort,* then we should talk positively to ourselves for trying to master the system and make our goals a reality. With every action, mental and physical that we take, we're creating beneficial *Experiences* that will have a lasting value and help heal whatever may be ailing us. To create beneficial *Experiences*, give them a lasting value by lengthening them, concentrating on them as they're happening. Really pay attention to them. Absorb them by sensing them sinking in to us. (These techniques are discussed at length in *Resilience*, p. 52-60).

🚫 Manage and control our *Emotions*. Practicing meditation and mindfulness will go a long way toward managing those *Emotions* of despair, depression, doubts, and dread that threaten to derail us.

Existentialism

An alternative system, *Existentialism* is a philosophical monster, a hydra with a controversial, perhaps ugly or even repulsive premise.

On 8/2/20, at 8:05 pm, while taking a break to watch a movie with my wife, my mind wandered into a very dark and dreary place: the abyss. I was suddenly overcome with dread. I lost my mindfulness and equanimity. My mind ran away from itself in fear: *Nothing matters anyway. Life is pointless. Who cares? What's the point? I might as well chuck it all, pack it in. I want ice cream and big meals of burgers, bread, pasta, pizza. Bowls of Kit Kat and Reese's cups. Potato chips. Nachos. The heck with it all. I'm going to end up failing. Regardless, I'll die someday. I'd rather die fat and happy, eating whatever I want, sleeping late, lying around watching TV.*

But I caught myself and expelled the negative thoughts by focusing on my breathing. I reverted to my mantras, my MS, my goals. I do NOT want all of that negative, self-destructive noise in my head and body.

So what caused my panic attack of doubt and despair? The lazy TV watching of a mediocre movie. Lying there like a brainless lump pushed me to the brink of the abyss. The movie and the watching of it was pointless, a waste of time, an obstacle to my progress. Yet, I sat there, paralyzed, allowing my mind to wallow in dread.

> *Watching a bad TV program, we become the TV program.*
> *We are what we feel and perceive.... We turn on the TV and*
> *leave it on, allowing someone else to guide us, shape us, and*
> *destroy us.... We must be aware which programs do harm*
> *to our nervous systems, minds, and hearts, and which pro-*
> *grams benefit us. (Hanh, pp. 13-14)*

Please don't misunderstand me: watching a *good* movie with my wife is not a waste of time. It's an important time spent with my love. But the good feelings of the warmth of holding my wife's hand and feeling her head on my shoulder were seriously negated by the horrible crap we were ingesting. We simply can't allow ourselves to waste our precious time on garbage. Garbage in, garbage out. So in paying attention, we have to continually ask ourselves: How much value is there for me in this current experience?

Being close to my wife is wonderful, but its value is severely lessened when the quality of what we're experiencing together is poor. The movie was vulgar and sophomoric, poorly written, mean-spirited, and flat out nasty. I felt like I was ingesting bowls of poisoned candy. Why subject myself to that crap? What it did was completely ruin what should have been a nice couple of hours with my wife. The rancid movie made me question my very existence: If this crap is considered good and I allow myself to watch it, what is the point of life, of anything? Why do movie studios make such garbage, who actually likes it, and what does that say about the state of humanity? Why was I so reluctant to simply say "this is crap" and stop watching it?

Well, I finally did tell my wife I hated it and she agreed. We surfed around, found something better to watch, and saved the night for ourselves.

But the point is, the rotten movie triggered feelings of dread, doubt, and despair. Negative in, negative out. So, what did I do mentally once we found a better viewing option? I reverted to my system. Took refuge in my mantras, MS, and goals. Deep breathing and mindfulness. That worked. I positively reinforced myself. Paying attention to what was bothering me dissipated the bother. Like when a deep pressure massage therapist presses hard on the source of a painful muscle to where it hurts so good the pain goes away.

Then, when I was by myself in my office later, my mindfulness restored, I recalled the dread and realized anew the promising application of **Existentialism** to this system.

"Emotion Recollected in Tranquility"

The Wordsworth once explained how he achieved the calm, soothing, mindful insightfulness of his lyrical ballads. He said that when he experienced a stimulating event or conversation that evoked a strong emotion—regardless of whether the experience was negative or positive—he would not immediately sit down with pen to paper. He would *not* try to write a poem while still in an agitated state. He would wait until his emotions settled and he'd regained a calm serenity by having distanced himself from the experience. Only then would he attempt to compose a poem, with the *"emotion recollected in tranquility."*

In that tranquil state, I recollected my strong emotion of dread earlier that evening. It got me to thinking about **Existentialism**. I've taught it many times in conjunction with 20th-century literature, primarily the life and works of Ernest Hemingway.

In essence, the premise of **Existentialism** is that life is meaningless. There is no God, no afterlife, nothing after we die. This meaningless existence is all there is. When we suffer the dread of doubt and despair, we're actually recognizing and realizing the truth. We've come to the brink of the abyss and have found ourselves staring down into the bottomless darkness.

Morbidly, yet interestingly enough, the final solution to both our life and our search for meaning is that we can always kill ourselves. However immediate and effective it may be, suicide is an unacceptable option. We simply must carry on. Life is too precious to give up on.

Once you realize that you have the power to end it all, you *also* have the power to keep living and make it mean something. Only you have the power to make your life meaningful. An existentialist, once deciding to live, lives his life according to a strict code. Hemingway's protagonists—Jake Barnes, Nick Adams, Santiago, to name a few—are called Code Heroes. To live your life despite this meaningless existence, you have to be a "code hero," committing to your own set of principles and goals, conducting yourself in a professional manner.

Clearly, the followers of *Existentialism* are the atheistic cousins of many otherwise like-minded men and women. If you believe in God, *Existentialism* is likely repulsive and disgusting to you. You believe that God *does* exist, that life *does* have meaning, that our time here on earth is *not* pointless, and we definitely *cannot* kill ourselves. But if you *don't* believe in God, then perhaps *Existentialism* is a perfect fit for you.

Relative to this **PEERLESS** system, I like the feeling it gives me—even if everything may be pointless and life meaningless and the dread real. That's our Waterloo there. Our moment of truth. Our O.K. Corral.

Ultimately and maybe on a daily basis, we have to fight the alcoholic's fight, knowing it's us or the booze, us or the pizza and brownie cookie, us next year or us today. That's what *Existentialism* teaches. The abyss is real. The dread is real. Life is, indeed, meaningless if you think it so. IF you—let's face it—ascribe to the atheistic world view, then life *is* meaningless. If there is no right and wrong, no good and evil, no God, no afterlife—or even the possibility of one—then what *is* it all about? What's the point of anything if there's no point to it all?

The point is life itself. Living is its own reason. If you have the power to end it all in an instant, or eat yourself to an early grave, then you also have the power to do the opposite: live as long as you can. You can do whatever you want. You can face the dreaded abyss and tell it to kiss off. You'll make your own meaning to your life by taking charge, making the decision to go down fighting and not whimpering.

> *Do not go gentle into that good night,*
>
> *Old age should burn and rave at close of day;*
>
> *Rage, rage against the dying of the light.*
>
> — *Dylan Thomas*

The existentialist commits to a positive, professional, stoic course. This **PEERLESS** system is just that: a highly professional, stoic program to positively impact our own lives. By taking charge, we walk back from the abyss and convert the dread into a calm hope for a better future—for as long as that future lasts. If we can kill ourselves, we can let ourselves live. We're in control—not the dread, not the doubts, not the nothingness. We have the power to turn our doubts into an indomitable faith in ourselves.

For more details about **Existentialism**, see my lecture: https://www.youtube.com/watch?v=R2Ja2w_ov8M&t=107s (The 11:50 mark is where the **Existentialism** discussion begins.)

Have faith in yourself. Bet on you. Take you to the bank. You can win if you think you can. *"Whether you think you can or you think you can't, you're right."* —Henry Ford.

Now that we've discussed getting our minds right, let's talk about feeding it reading.

CHAPTER 4

Read

"The difference between where you are today

and where you'll be five years from now

will be found in the quality of books you've read."

– Jim Rohn

"The more that you read, the more things you will know.

The more that you learn, the more places you'll go."

– Dr. Seuss

You might think it's odd I'm talking about reading. Maybe I just couldn't think of another word to pick for the letter R. But no. Reading is essential to upgrade and supercharge your chances for optimum success in life.

Bias Alert Right off the bat, I'll tell you that I love reading. Period. It feels so good. I grew up reading books. I've read thousands and thousands of books. I taught reading and writing from 1976-2015. Roughly 10 years in high school and 30 in college. That was my entire professional career and I loved it.

As I'm writing this book, I'm in my office lined with books. I love books. I love words. I love the act of reading, the connection with the writers, the stimulation of the ideas, the way the words signify thoughts and convey meaning. The magic of being right there inside the writer's mind as he or she wrote the words 10, 50, 100, even 500 years ago.

Words, books, stories make writers almost immortal. They live again every time someone reads their words. When we read, we're engaging in a conversation with the writer of the book. Our minds actively think and talk to the book, annotate mentally or even physically by writing in the margins or keeping notes on a pad or in a GDoc. We pause and think, ruminate over the words, reread them, ask questions, wonder about them. We talk to the writers. It's magical and miraculous. Words are thoughts in writers' minds.

What came first: words or thoughts? How do we think if not in words? Words are what make us human. As Descartes rightly posited, *"I think, therefore I am."* Did humans even exist prior to words? After all, in the beginning was the Word.

What Should We Read?

I started to say "anything and everything," but no. That's not great advice. Not at all. With our limited time and an almost infinite number (it may as well be infinite because we have zero chance of ever reading everything) of books, articles, blogs to choose from, we must be highly selective in our choices for reading matter. We need to carefully curate our reading.

🎞 Make a list of what you want to read.

I'd start by not counting websites, surfing the internet on your phone, news, blogs, etc. They don't count. In fact, they might be counterproductive to your mindfulness, calm, and attention to what's truly important (See Chapter 3, Equanimity). Refer to Ferriss's "low information diet." The words produced by the media and SM are predominantly negative time wasters, like junk food or fear-mongering sensationalism. They will very likely not advance your goals or fill your mind and heart with positive thoughts of any personal value. Since I've reduced my intake of these types of words, I've felt more at peace, more calm and hopeful, and been more productive, attentive, and mindful. Everything in *PEERLESS* has been enhanced and advanced at a steadier pace and greater effectiveness than weeks ago when I was surfing news and SM for hours a day.

So, what sort of books and articles should you be reading? How about self-improvement, motivational, mindfulness books? Novels are fun and can sharpen the saw and be relaxing and such. But right now, I don't think they're a priority to read. And that statement is coming from a 40-year teacher of literature. From Goethe to Vonnegut, Shakespeare to Hawthorne, Twain, Melville, Chopin, Hemingway, Faulkner, O'Conner, and Hurston, from Voltaire, Camus, Brecht, and Rousseau to Marquez, Shaw, Thomas, Angelou, and Frost—I've taught hundreds of different authors and their books, stories and poetry. There's little in this world or life—other than my family and baseball—that I love and cherish more than literature. But right now, my life is laser-beam focused on self-improvement, better health, and becoming peerless. Therefore, I need to read non-fiction books and articles that teach, support, and guide me in my quest to create a better me.

📖 Using the 🌐 symbol, I've referred to, quoted, and recommended many relevant books. Many more exist. Browse the non-fiction, self-help, diet, exercise, philosophy, longevity, anti-aging, science (and other) sections at your local brick-and-mortar bookstore. Online sites are good, but you can't hold the books, feel their heft and bend their spine, put your nose in the pages and breathe in the wonderful smell. Besides, Amazon doesn't need your money. Your local bookstore does.

I would also highly recommend poetry. If you already "get" poetry, great. If you don't "get" it or like it, take heart: now's the time and I'm the teacher to help you learn to love it. Poetry will soothe and inspire you like no other reading. Poetry is a mantra in verse. I could go on, but I've already said it best years ago in a lecture for my college students: https://www.youtube.com/watch?v=Ukc9OIQHqqA&t=7s.

When Should We Read?

All the livelong day. Whenever you're not doing anything else related to this system. When you're not sleeping, eating, writing, or exercising, you should be reading. I suppose you need to spend some time with your spouse or significant other and your kids. That can't be helped. Just kidding. Loving thy family is #1. But whenever possible, read. Do NOT waste time on SM, watching TV, or any other former (I hope) activities that merely spin your wheels or masquerade as important things to do with your precious time.

Where Should We Read?

Everywhere and anywhere. I keep different books on the sofa, in my office, on my nightstand, and in my car—just so I never don't have one nearby because I forgot to grab it. Having books all over the place also reminds us to read them! I read at the beach and in the car as I'm parked against the fence watching my son's baseball practice. (I don't read during his games—too important and fun and valuable to watch).

Why Should We Read?

We have brains we need to exercise. We have knowledge we need to acquire. We have goals that the books we read will help us achieve. Reading is a relaxing, mindful, critical activity for our mental health.

Many studies have scientifically proven that reading can significantly slow cognitive decline.

> *Mental activities like reading and writing can preserve structural integrity in the brains of older people, according to a new study presented today at the annual meeting of the Radiological Society of North America (RSNA). The study*

included 152 elderly participants, mean age 81 years, from the Rush Memory and Aging Project, a large-scale study looking at risk factors for Alzheimer's disease. Participants underwent brain MRI using a 1.5-T scanner within one year of clinical evaluation. The researchers collected anatomical and DTI data and used it to generate diffusion anisotropy maps.

Data analysis revealed significant associations between the frequency of cognitive activity in later life and higher diffusion anisotropy values in the brain. "Several areas throughout the brain, including regions quite important to cognition, showed higher microstructural integrity with more frequent cognitive activity in late life," said Dr. Konstantinos Arfanakis. "Keeping the brain occupied late in life has positive outcomes." ("Reading, Writing, and Playing Games May Help Aging Brains Stay Healthy," rush.edu, 11/26/12)

In the Health and Retirement Study conducted by researchers at Yale University School of Public Health, an ongoing investigation of 5635 people who were 50 or older *"determined that people who read books regularly had a 20% lower risk of dying over the next 12 years compared with people who weren't readers or who read periodicals"* ("Reading Books").

In yet another study,

...researchers tested almost 300 older adults' memory and thinking ability every year for 6 years...After the participants' deaths (at an average age of 89), the researchers examined their brains for evidence of the physical signs of dementia, which typically include lesions, plaques, and neural tangles, the brain abnormalities often associated with memory lapses. Those people who reported that they read were protected against brain lesions and tangles and

self-reported memory decline over the 6-year study. In addition, remaining an avid reader into old age reduced memory decline by more than 30%, compared to engaging in other forms of mental activity. Those who read the most had the fewest physical signs of dementia.... (Castle)

The evidence is conclusive: reading can definitely extend your life.

How Should We Read?

Fast or slow, skim or every word, taking notes, stopping, pausing, or plowing straight ahead? You should read however you've always read, but better. Engage. Concentrate. Read with faith and Purpose. If you need to speed up, skim, skip paragraphs or even chapters, okay. Make those decisions. You're the boss of your reading. But definitely annotate by marking up, underlining, putting brackets around important lines, highlighting. Make sure your reading time is maximized by paying attention and always be evaluating the applications for yourself. How is this information helping me? How can I use it?

Personally, I annotate and evaluate like crazy. If I'm learning and making connections to my life while I'm reading, then it's truly exciting. It's an experience, an event, a happening.

My reading takes two forms: 1) the initial reading and annotating; and 2) at another time, after I've finished the book, I sit at my PC and go back through it, entering my annotated notes into a Gdoc for each book. I have a Gdoc specifically entitled "Book Reviews" in which I record all of a book's highlights, complete with quotation marks and parenthetical page numbers. Documentation is a good thing. I've turned many of my rough draft review notes into full-fledged book reviews that I've posted on my Edit911 website and blasted out in SM (Facebook, Twitter, Linkedin). The practice helps my website with new, fresh, informative content that's not necessarily on brand; that is, it doesn't matter if the book and its review has anything to do with editing or an editing service. It's just good information for my clients and potential clients. I really don't care if it generates more business. It's what I read that's good and I want to make my positive review available to my reading public. Period. Share and share alike. Pay it forward.

Want Some Help to Read Better or Faster?

There are many online resources to help you become a better reader, but one of the best is Jim Kwik's. He's developed an effective system for not only reading faster but reading with more comprehension and retention: https://kwiklearning.com.

Supplemental Rs

Reinvigorate, Refresh, Restore, Recharge, Relax. I find that reading does all of those things for me, but if you don't and even if you do, find other activities to "sharpen the saw" as Covey calls the process of recharging your batteries. Several times a day—or whenever you feel yourself slipping— Recharge and Refocus by Repeating your mantras.

At this very moment (8/1/20, 2:00 PM), my son and I are at Cocoa Beach. He surfs while I body surf. The sun is recharging me. It is extremely reinvigorating and refreshing. The saltwater soothes and restores health to my skin.

The ocean and poetry are one and the same—rhythmic, universal, timeless. For me, there's no better combination to make me feel alive, to inspire me than to read poetry at the beach. Take Walt Whitman's classic *Leaves of Grass* to the beach. He's America's greatest poet, a transcendental treasure trove of magnificent, soaring verse:

As I ebb'd with the ocean of life,

As I wended the shores I know,

As I walk'd where the ripples continually wash you Paumanok,

Where they rustle up hoarse and sibilant,

Where the fierce old mother endlessly cries for her castaways,

I musing late in the autumn day, gazing off southward,

Held by this electric self out of the pride of which I utter poems,

Was seiz'd by the spirit that trails in the lines underfoot,

The rim, the sediment that stands for all the water and all the land of the globe.

(from "As I Ebb'd With the Ocean of Life")

Should you care to know more about Whitman, here's my lecture: https://www.youtube.com/watch?v=5h9gpQCHnX0&t=6s.

If you're not yet an aficionado of poetry, perhaps it would help to hear someone read some great poetry aloud. This video reading of some of his poetry (along with Emily Dickinson's) may help you appreciate his greatness: https://www.youtube.com/watch?v=H3l3dqcClhQ&t=8s).

Whitman's appreciation of the ocean is shared by his contemporary Thoreau, whose words I recall while I'm standing on the shore, breathing deeply: "*I am sensible that I am imbibing good health when I open my mouth to the wind.*"

I'm getting exercise and I'm getting much-needed time with my son and having fun. Fun is essential. And this is one of the main ways I have fun: coming to the beach.

Take a Risk. Let what you're reading challenge you to take risks. Following this system may be a risk, but isn't it worth it?

Take Responsibility. The more you read, the more responsible you are becoming for your own existence and the more you realize the importance of responsibility. Ultimately, you are responsible for you and everything that happens to you. Short of a tragedy out of the blue, you manage your future.

☞ <u>Be Resilient.</u> You have to be able to bounce back every single day. Reading also teaches resiliency. Sometimes, reading may have the effect of making you feel like it's impossible because there's so much to learn and so much to do and so many people know more than you do. But that's a reactive reaction, if you will. Be resilient and bounce back to learn more from your reading. Be resilient to realize that the more you read, the more you know, and the more possibilities open up for you.

CHAPTER 5

Learn

"These fragments I have shored against my ruins"
—T.S. Eliot, <u>The Waste Land and Other Poems</u>

"Live as if you were to die tomorrow. Learn as if you were to live forever."
— *Mahatma Gandhi*

It's *all* about learning, isn't it?

Whenever people have asked me what I learned while studying for my Ph.D. I always answer: *"I learned how little I know."* Back in the day, my main assignment was to read. The library was my home base, not the internet. It existed in 1988-1993 (my doctoral study years), but I have zero citations or references from the internet in my published papers and dissertation. I lived in the library and in the pages of books, primarily learning about the extent of my ignorance. We can never let up on learning.

Why Should We Learn?

To enhance our ability to succeed in achieving our goals.

The incomparable Tony Robbins trademarked his CANI system, which stands for *"Constant And Never-ending Improvement."* He says, *"I believe that the level of success we experience in life is in direct proportion to the level of our commitment to CANI"* (Robbins, p. 96).

To improve our lives, improve our selves, and live longer: *"Learning is the superpower of superpowers, the one that grows the rest of them. If you want to stipend your growth curve, it pays to learn about learning"* (Resilient, p. 50).

Essentially, constant learning is good for your cognitive functioning. And what's good for the brain is good for our goodness.

> *There's a saying in brain science based on the work of Donald Hebb: "**Neurons that fire together wire together.**" **The more they fire together, the more they wire together.** In essence, you develop psychological resources by having sustained and repeated experiences of them that are turned into durable changes in your brain. You become more grateful, confident, or determined by repeatedly installing experiences of gratitude, confidence, or determination. Similarly, you center yourself increasingly in the Responsive green zone—with an underlying sense of peace, contentment, and love—by having an internalizing many experiences of safety, satisfaction, and connection.* (Resilient, p. 50)

Learning makes us better people. And learning is a synergistic activity: a busy brain is a healthy brain is a learning brain, and a brain can only be healthy when it is active. *"By failing to engage it in intellectually challenging activities, your brain will fail to grow new connections, and it will indeed become disorganized and ultimately dysfunctional"* (Transcend, p. 8).

Learning From Life-Changing Events

When my twin daughters were born it was a William Wordsworthian event for me. His line *"The Child is father of the Man"* implied more about how acquiring a childlike sense of wonder of the world gives birth to and empowers a maturity, a growth into actual adulthood. Yet, poetry's wonderful magic is its ambiguity and how we can see other meanings applicable to ourselves. So, in that case, I took it to mean that the birth of my children was the birth of my adulthood. I finally grew up on that day. I finally became a man and realized that being a father demanded I leave behind some of my former flaws and irresponsible behavior.

How to Learn?

An old friend of mine had a standard comeback when someone confronted him or argued with him about something. And that happened a lot because he was a drunk. The nicest, smartest, most charming guy you ever met. But a drunk. So he was a magnet for trouble. Myself, other friends, his mother, brother, strangers—he regularly pissed off all of us by his irresponsible, ridiculous behavior. When we called him out on it—being late, forgetting commitments, sloughing off our plans—he'd just look at us with his wry, disarming, half-drunk smile and say, "Teach me to learn."

I always thought it was funny and just his standard bullshit. But now, I wonder. Maybe it was, in fact, a subconscious acknowledgment that he just couldn't learn how to function as sober people do.

Assuming we're sober, we can learn. But it shouldn't be assumed that learning is easy or automatic.

Rick Hanson has developed his own HEAL process that teaches us *how to learn.*

You can guide the structure-building processes of your brain in four steps, which I summarize with the acronym HEAL:

Activation

1. *Have a beneficial experience: notice it or create it.*

Installation

2. *Enrich it: Stay with it, feeling it fully.*

3. *Absorb it: receive it into yourself.*

4. *Link it (optional): use it to soothe and replace painful, harmful psychological material.*

There it is. Hanson has brilliantly, concisely explained exactly *how to learn* with his acronym HEAL. It's so simple, really. It starts with being wide awake, self-reliant, and disciplined. Be tuned in. Focus. Pay Attention. Practice Mindful Meditation (see Chapter 3), and use RAS. Why these learning skills and strategies aren't taught in our schools is beyond me. Perhaps they are, bit by bit, here and there, by various teachers. But there should be a mandatory, core curriculum class entitled *"How to Learn"* or *"Learning 101."*

At any rate, there it is. It's all there for us. All the skills we need, laid out in HEAL and developed later in this book.

Progressive Mastery

Brendon Burchard's system of "Progressive Mastery" (PM) is brilliant in its simplicity and common sense. All about structure, habitual behavior, and persistence, PM is an elegant formulation of how best to get good at anything by following a set of 10 steps—including setting "stretch goals," attaching "emotion and meaning" to them, identifying "factors critical to success," visualizing, and measuring your progress.

> *Perhaps the three best findings of contemporary research tell us that you can get better at practically anything if you keep a growth mindset (the belief that you can improve with effort), focus on your goals with passion and perseverance, and practice with excellence.* (Burchard, p. 206)

What to Learn

Anything you want. Refer back to your SSI & MIL. What do you know and want to know more about? What *don't* you know that you'd like to know?

🖳 If you haven't already, brainstorm and make a list of everything you'd like to learn. Want to be a better fisherman, carpenter, mechanic, salesman, father, husband, mother, son, daughter, friend, dancer, lover? Your teachers are out there by the tens of thousands in books, articles, websites, and YouTube videos. Or you could consider taking a college or trade school class or two locally or online.

One of my twin daughters—the free-spirit, freelancer, world traveler (been to 46 countries)—bought a fixer-upper house a few years ago. When I walked into it, I was shocked. I thought she'd made a terrible mistake. It was a complete mess. I mean nothing in it was okay. The repair or replace list was total. The floors, ceiling, walls, cabinets, stairs, windows, appliances, roof, gutter, pool, screen enclosure, driveway, yard—everything had to be repaired or replaced.

"*How can you afford to pay for all these repairs?*" I asked her. "*I'm not paying anybody to do anything. I'm going to do it all myself,*" she replied. And she did.

With her own two hands and grit, and the help of YouTube videos, she replaced windows, the pool enclosure screens and some bent beams, all the floors with new laminate and even marble in one bathroom, all the appliances (she had them delivered but installed them herself), including a new water heater, shingles on the roof, several strips of gutters, and all the yard work (lawn and hedges, removing wasp nests along the way). She plastered, sawed, mitered, grouted, mixed, laid, removed, installed, troubleshot, solved every problem, and completely—I mean 95%–remodeled the entire 3000sf house all by herself. What a woman. And she's single, guys. She's quite a catch. Good luck, though. She wants the "perfect" man or she'll remain single. She's broken hearts along her do-it-yourself path around the world. At any rate, what woman needs a man when she's got YouTube?

🎬 YouTube videos are a great resource. If you're interested in reading, writing, or literature topics, check out my site: https://www.youtube.com/feed/my_videos.

Make Time to Learn

Move learning to Quadrant #1 in your time management matrix. It's important and urgent. *"High performers are very clear about the skill sets they need to develop now to win in the future....They tend to have more blocks of time already scheduled for learning then do their peers....they built a **curriculum** for themselves and are actively engaged in learning"* (**Burchard, p. 71).**

☞ **PEERLESS is a "curriculum" I made for myself. I hope it's giving you ideas also.**

🎬 Now it's time to get back to working on our bodies!

CHAPTER 6

Exercise

"Those who think they have no time for bodily exercise
will sooner or later have to find time for illness."
—Edward Stanley (1826-1893)

"If you're in an older demographic, exercise is everything. It's been
shown to be as effective for depression as medications....It also helps
boost serotonin production and improves sleep....It decreases pain
and reduces anxiety...."
—Brendon Burchard (p. 119)

We have to keep our bodies moving and our muscles toned or else. Our hearts need the cardio. Our spirits need the mojo, the endorphins, the feel-good feeling of looking good.

> *According to WHO, sedentary lifestyles increase all causes*
> *of mortality, double the risk of cardiovascular diseases,*
> *diabetes, and obesity, and increase the risks of colon can-*
> *cer, high blood pressure and more serious health conditions.*
> *("Sedentary Lifestyle")*

Are you a couch-potato? Do you sit a lot watching TV, or even at work on a computer or doing other work-related tasks?

*A growing body of evidence suggests that **spending too many hours sitting is hazardous to your health.** Habitual inactivity raises risks for obesity, diabetes, cardiovascular disease, deep-vein thrombosis, and metabolic syndrome.... Given the research, breaking up long blocks of sitting to flex your muscles seems like a wise move for all of us, so try to build more activity into your day. Set a timer to remind you to get up and move around every so often. Take your phone calls standing up. Try an adjustable standing desk for your computer. Instead of sitting in an armchair while watching TV, sit on a stability ball, which makes you use your muscles to stay upright. And, yes, do our joint pain relief exercises. ("The Dangers of Sitting")*

Dr. Gundry takes a deep dive into exactly how exercise benefits the body:

Exercise is another perfect example of hormesis—limited stressors you put on your body to make yourself stronger. Like other examples of hormetic stressors such as caloric restriction, exercise stimulates autophagy, the recycling of old, worn out cellular components, and a similar process called the unfolded protein response (UPR). In the case of UPR, the cell degrades dysfunctional misfolded proteins, restoring the health of the cell. (p. 133)

Mike Matthews also makes a convincing case for exercise:

Workouts build more than muscle. They build character. *They teach us how to have the courage to commit to goals....how to create purpose and meaning.... how to stop making excuses....how to get gritty and push through pain* *and adversity....how to value long-term satisfaction over immediate gratification. If we have the power to change our bodies, we have the power to change our lives. (Matthews, pp. 36-37).*

Here's the kicker: exercise is also good for your brain.

Exercise increases production of brain derived neurotrophic factor BDNF. BDNF causes new neurons to grow in your hippocampus and other areas in your brain, creating increased plasticity and ability to learn faster, remember more and improve overall brain function. (Burchard, p. 117)

Before You Start an Exercise Program Consult With Your Doctor

Make an appointment with your physician. Ask her for the most comprehensive physical on her menu. Tell her you want to get in the best physical shape of your life and you need to know if anything—anything at all—is wrong with you or could possibly be improved by better diet, supplements, and/or exercise.

Among other questions, ask your doctor if you can safely exert yourself. If so, how much? Ask about your heart and your back. Tell her what sort of exercise you do now. Assess what kind of shape you're currently in. Discuss what your goals are.

Answer all those questions and make yourself a fitness plan.

Where Should You Exercise?

Inside and outside. At home, you can do pushups, sit-ups, any number of exercises. Ride a bike, swim in a pool or at the beach. Run if you can. If you can't, jog or walk.

I prefer a gym.

Join A Gym

*"A refuge from the chaos around us, a world of a room that we can
create to satisfy dreams and desires, providing us with principles,
values and standards, a game worth playing. Without a game worth
playing, nothing else really matters."*

– Michael Matthews (p. 39)

"My gym is how I get refocused."

–Tim McGraw (from Ferriss, Tools, p. 465)

I'm not alone in believing that a gym is essential—unless, of course, you
create your own home gym. Only do so if you have the room and the extra
discipline to faithfully use the equipment. Tom Brady's book, *The TB12
Method,* and website detail a home gym based primarily on bands, that he
conveniently sells. Two of the most popular machine-based home gyms are
Nordic Trak and Bowflex. Here's an independent site that compares them:
https://bestreviews.com/best-home-gyms.

However, I much prefer and highly recommend going to a real gym. You
get out of the house. It's a place to go with like-minded, motivated people
around you. You can discreetly observe how others do their workouts, put
in their work. Much more conducive to working hard than at home, where
it's just you, and whatever distractions come up.

If you've never been to a gym, go now. Find a good gym and consult with
their trainer about your goals.

Questions to Ask a Trainer

Check out 2-3 gyms in your area. Hopefully, there are some. Call them
and book a tour. Ask them specifically for a private, introductory consult

with their trainer. Tell the trainer about your health concerns and workout goals. Then ask the trainer these specific questions:

1. Tell me about yourself. Do you have any certifications?

2. How many days a week should I work out?

3. What should I eat before and after a workout?

4. What are the best exercises to do to address my specific body issues; e.g. stomach, hips, arms, etc.?

5. How much one-on-one training will you be available to give me?

6. Should I do cardio or weights first?

7. What are some diet and supplement recommendations?

These questions and your time together should give you a good feel for whether and how much this trainer will be able to assist you in creating and sticking to a program. If the trainer doesn't actually offer to *train* you much at all, I'd consider the gym with a trainer that *does* seem enthusiastic about *training* you—at least at the outset.

How to Pick a Gym That's Right for You

I don't see a great deal of difference among gyms besides ambiance, hours, cost, location, and trainers. Most of them have all the machines and free weights you need to get in a good workout. If you want convenient hours and location, it's an easy call. If personal training and a variety of small group classes are important to you, then by all means use that as a selection criteria. If you're concerned with the "type" of people who are members and how the gym "feels" to you, then try to visit it a few times to get a sample size of those concerns before committing to join it. If it's about cost, Planet Fitness can't be beat: $10 a month, or $24 if you want the Black Card membership, which comes with massage chairs, tanning beds, discounts on merch and drinks, and free guest privileges.

Once you make your choice and join a gym, get with the trainer you already interviewed. He or she can set you up with a program of machines and weights to suit your needs.

The gym is a great refuge. Make it your 2nd home. Where you're able to focus and pay strict attention to the task at hand: your 30 or 45 or 60-minute workout. You'll grow to love coming to your gym!

Books & Websites to Check Out

There are hundreds, of course, but here are 4 of my favorites.

Tom Brady's TB12 Method: How to Do What You Love, Better and For Longer

Tom needs no introduction. He's proven himself to be an expert in staying fit. At 45 years old, he's now with the Tampa Bay Bucs and vowing—some say—to play until he's 50. A 7-time Super Bowl champion Quarterback, Tom founded TB12, a full-service fitness company with books, a complete home training program, training equipment, supplements, physical gyms, and numerous videos, podcasts, email tips, and more.

His book is big and beautifully laid out with hundreds of pictures detailing dozens of specific exercises—many with bands he sells on his website—that you can do at home. The section on Nutrition includes many recipes with full-color pictures of delicious dishes. It's a Tom-Terrific production that's fun and easy to read or skim through. A real page-turner.

Here's just one of many 5-star reviews on Amazon:

This book is a summary of Brady's healthy lifestyle and exercise routine. As a nurse practitioner trained as a Certified Strength and Conditioning Specialist, I found his beliefs to be pretty well grounded in science and commonly accepted practices and enjoyed the content. It is comprehensive and well-thought out. It's his way of telling his story and then thoroughly covering all aspects of life that lead to achieving a lifetime of sustained peak performance that makes it unique. If we all did what he suggests, we'd all be fit, healthy, and happier. If coaches followed these guidelines, we'd have less injuries nationwide. It should be required reading of all high school athletes and especially the coaches who still don't get it.

As you might imagine, his website is also world-class excellent: https:// tb12sports.com/. His store is a one-stop fitness shopping mecca, even offering online training options.

<u>Tim Ferriss *The 4-Hour Body*</u>

Another industry heavyweight, Ferriss's book is also massive and comprehensive. Unlike Brady's book, there are no pretty full-color pictures, however. Tom probably had a blank check from Simon & Shuster. Regardless, Tim's book is also loaded with black and white pictures of exercises, and the copy is extensive. He has sections on everything from "Subtracting Fat" (with details of his own specific diet to do so) and "Adding Muscle" to "Improving Sex," "Perfecting Sleep," and "Getting Stronger." Tim's writing style is hyper-lively and fun. He's got stories and charts and tables and quotes for everything. The guy is a walking encyclopedia.

Tim's rogue and rambling style—in writing, lifestyle, and the ideas in this book—is definitely different. He can be all over the map and apparently his methods don't work for everybody. Here are excerpts from two negative and one positive Amazon review:

As much as I like the "rogue science" approach of the book, being a health scientist myself, I'm currently on the diet that this book talks about, have been for almost 3 weeks, and haven't lost even 1% body fat.

Tim Ferriss is excellent when it comes to productivity, business, marketing and interviewing. Physical fitness - look elsewhere. Not everything requires a 'hack.' Sometimes, the conventional methods + hard work will equal great results!

There is a wealth of information in this book, and it has helped me lose weight, gain strength and run faster in the last 12 months. Like most of Ferriss' work, it could easily be misunderstood. Be clear that it isn't about shortcuts or 'hacks,' it's about efficiently getting maximum benefit from the minimum input - but that 'minimum input' still requires effort and dedication. You'll get out what you're prepared to put in.

Tim's website can't be beat. Exhibiting an astoundingly impressive amount of energy and knowledge, Tim covers a broader array of topics than anyone else that I know of. Check out the unmatched number and quality of his podcast interviews: https://tim.blog/.

Michael Matthews *Bigger, Leaner, Stronger* (for men) & *Thinner, Leaner, Stronger* (for women)

Two terrific books, they are both no-nonsense guides to eating right and exercising efficiently to lose weight and body fat, and gain muscle. Citing dozens of solid research and programs, Mike's books are a fast, easy read, with very specific and effective tips and plans for dieting and exercising. He's probably a very unpopular guy in the diet, exercise, and supplement industries because he's extremely critical of them, debunking and condemning many assorted popular dieting and exercising methods, programs, and supplements.

Here are 4 excellent and 2 not-so-good Amazon reviews—three for each book:

> *Obsessed with this book. To the point I've accomplished little else while reading it and simultaneously listening to the audible version. Yes I'm that girl. Didn't want to miss anything!!! Everything he says is ON POINT.*

> *You can literally buy this book and trash every single copy of Shape, Oxygen, and Cosmo you have, discontinue the crazy dangerous CrossFit, and kiss Jillian Michaels goodbye. I've seen it, done it, plus 20 years in the Army, many marathons and two babies later determined that these do not work. Michael Matthew' book does!*

> *I bought this book because of all the great reviews and I honestly didn't even read the entire book because it was so repetitive and boring. I found the information mediocre at best. Maybe some information useful but not much.*

> *At the risk of being dramatic, this book and its author's online content basically changed my life. By opening my eyes and showing me just how simple (I said simple, not easy) weight loss is if you put in the work and practice some willpower. Using the methods in this book, i was able to lose 109 lbs. and as of today have maintained this body for 2 years now.*

> *Great book. This guy tells it straight. Training, supplementation, mind-set. He even tells you when it's his personal view or when the science leaves the picture unclear. He cites many sources - both those that support other views and those that support his own. Knowledge is power they say and if you want to REALLY, TRUELY know how to get stronger and*

build muscle, this book empowers by giving you all the details and studies to become informed.

I'm shocked I got through the introduction without closing out of the book and hitting "Remove From Device". It is basically a 300-page infomercial. Mike, buddy, pal... we bought the book. You closed the deal. Continuing to bash us over the head with your "What if I told you's or headlining sections promising SECRETS is just unnecessary. We're in. You have our money.

Mike's website is also loaded with articles, blogs, podcasts, a store, and more. Good source of information about all things fitness-related: https://legionathletics.com/michael-matthews/.

<u>Zuby Strong Advice</u>

Very interesting, multi-talented Englishman, Zuby is an Oxford graduate, rapper, podcast host, and bodybuilder. His book is very good: concise, motivational, practical, and entertaining. Unfortunately, it's not available in hard copy or on Amazon. It's only available as a pdf or audiobook on his website.

Here are 2 reviews. They're from his own website, but I agree with them.

The book is written how all instructional books should be written. Short, simple, and to the point. I'm 51 years old and only 6 months into this journey and I am already in the best shape I've ever been in. I've always been too lazy exercise, but this book will teach you that being in shape is actually relatively simple. Zuby covers being mentally prepared, how to eat depending on whether you want to gain or lose weight, and then how to train.

Most people don't know where to start on the road to getting fit. They get intimidated by all these crazy workouts and spartan diets. Zuby really simplifies this with common sense and basic nutritional advice that anyone can apply to their daily life. If you can't apply it, what good is it. Worth every penny.

Like the man, Zuby's website—and book and music—are worth checking out: https://www.zubymusic.com/.

What Exercises Should We Do?

I start by stretching my spine, back, shoulders, hamstrings. Lots of stretches, standing and sitting on the floor. Then I work my upper body one day and legs the next. Fairly simple.

As always—here we go again—there's wide disagreement about how much and what exact type of exercises to do.

Cardio & Aerobic

Some say lots of cardio and aerobic training; others say not so much. Asprey is representative of those who warn that too much *"raises the cortisol (stress hormone) level, which causes inflammation and accelerates aging....it is well-established that excessive aerobic exercise can cause oxidative stress"* (*Game Changers*, pp. 162-163). *"Too much,"* from what I've been able to deduce, is more than 20 minutes, 3x a week. Keep it to that and we're good. Any more than that and we're stressing ourselves out.

Strength Training

Strength Training is weightlifting and the various machines (such as *Cybex*) that work individual parts of your body one at a time. Personally, I love those machines. Very smooth and safe and reliably accurate. I set them at my preferred weight and go to work. The consensus advice is that we should set them at the highest weight at which we can manage to do 3 sets of 8-10 reps. We should strain and push ourselves to do those 3 sets of 8-10 reps. They should not be easy. We should really struggle, grit our teeth, and feel our muscles burn. In that way, we know we're doing maximum good and building muscle mass and strength—which, according to studies, are the two *"most important parameters"* that could predict aging. *"These markers outranked cholesterol level, high blood pressure, resting heart rate, maximum heart rate, and all other factors as predictors of healthy aging"* (Asprey, *Game Changers*, p. 163).

Let's read that again, slowly. The importance of that statement cannot be overemphasized. **The most important measure of our chances of aging well is how strong and muscular we are.** Ergo, the importance of getting to a gym and working out.

Movement

Simply moving is the simplest, most profoundly effective exercise of all. Without regular, consistent and persistent movement, our bodies stagnate and degenerate. Low-level movement, such as bike riding, walking, and simply (there it is again: it's simple) getting up from our chairs, taking a break every 15 to 20 minutes from whatever it is we're doing (whether it's working at our desks our watching TV), and moving around and stretching is essential.

> *All forms of conscious movement lead to a cascade of effects that stimulate neurogenesis (the birth of new neurons), neuroprotection, neuroregeneration, cell survival, synaptic plasticity, and the formation and retention of new memories. Moving also makes you happier, most likely because it stimulates the release of endorphins.* (Asprey, *Game Changers*, p. 165)

What Should We Do After Exercising?

Recovery. Rest those muscles you worked out. To aid your muscles in recovering, repairing, and growing, be sure to take a good BCAA (Branched Chain Amino Acids) powder that contains as its main ingredient L-Leucine. *"Of the 20 different amino acids, only leucine can activate a gene transcription factor, mammalian target rapamycin (mTOR), which increases protein synthesis in your muscles, and therefore helps build muscle and prevent the loss of muscle as you age"* (Asprey, *Game Changers*, p. 179). (We'll be discussing mTOR a lot more in Chapter 8). You should also take a Glutamine supplement powder. Exercising depletes your body's store of this amino acid that, like leucine, is essential in muscle recovery and growth. They both come in various flavors that make a delicious post-workout drink when mixed in water. Your local GNC or health food store has them both in powder form.

What if I'm Losing Weight Dieting but Not Gaining or Even Losing Muscle?

This problem of losing weight but not gaining or even losing muscle is very common. I initially suffered from it until I researched it and learned some things. To lose fat and weight, we need to restrict calories and force the body to burn our existing fat. Unfortunately, the body also burns muscle unless we do something to stop it.

To gain muscle, our bodies need to be in a state of caloric surplus that gives us the energy it takes to repair and grow those bigger muscles.

So how do we achieve those two conflicting goals at the same time?

- Save calories by reducing carbs.

- Exercise smarter. More weight, fewer reps. For example, rather than doing 3 sets of 12 reps at 75 pounds, do 3 sets of 5-7 reps at 100 pounds. More weight equals more muscle tear and burn and recovery and growth.

- Give your muscle groups a day off between working them. Don't do the same muscles two days in a row. Do upper body one day, lower body the next, and so on.

- Increase your protein. This aspect deserves to be repeated and emphasized.

More Protein!

There's no substitute for protein when it comes to building muscle. It's the #1 nutrient for creating new tissue. When cutting calories, never cut them from sources of protein. Many studies have shown that we can restrict our caloric intake and still gain muscle *if* we eat enough protein.

So, the question is: How much protein should we get each day? There's so much debate about how much protein we should have it's almost ridiculous. The more I research, the more I find "experts" disagreeing. Some say "too much" is unhealthy and set a very low amount as the daily intake, such as .2 grams of protein for every pound you weigh. For a 200 pound man that's just 40 grams. That's the low end. The average is .4, which is 80 grams. But the ones tackling the weight loss vs. muscle gain issue argue that as much as 1.5 is safe. For a 200 pound man, that's 300 grams of protein a day. Is that dangerous? Although it's rare to develop a disease from too much protein, massive amounts *can* harm your kidneys or lead to heart disease. More common, less harmful side effects are constipation, diarrhea, and bad breath.

The obvious dilemma, a real balancing act, is that 100 grams of protein equate to approximately 400 calories. So if you have 300 grams, that's 1200 calories just in protein. Which is why we should start slowly in increasing our protein intake, monitor its effects, and adjust accordingly.

I currently (9/20/20) weigh 205 pounds and aim for 200 grams a day. I start with 50 in the morning in a protein shake. Then I go from there to get to the 200 mark with my food and more shakes if necessary. If all is well and my blood work at my yearly physical checks out, I'm going to increase it to 250-300 grams per day.

🎬 As I always caution, I'm not a doctor, so don't take my advice without doing your own homework.

A Plug for a Special, Very Cool "Nerd Fitness Expert" Website

Check this site out: https://www.nerdfitness.com. Steve Kamb's site is smart, funny, fast, and gives great advice about all-things-fitness (eating and exercise). It's just plain fun and brilliant. And no, just like with WW, I have zero connection with the guy. I just find him and his site to be super cool and informative.

Grow Your Expectation for Excellence

That's really what we're striving for here with **PEERLESS**: expecting ourselves to be excellent.

"Human excellence is a state of mind." —Socrates

We're not kids, but many studies of kids' academic achievement have concluded that one of the main factors responsible for their high grades is having had parents who *expected* them to be *excellent*. Doug Lemov, the author of *Teach Like a Champion*, states that *"One consistent finding of academic research is that high expectations are the most reliable driver of high student achievement, even in students who do not have a history of successful achievement"* (p. 1).

The same goes for us: we greatly enhance our chances of getting what we aim for when we have a MS, Goals, Action Plans, and a system to keep us eating and exercising right. So we need to stay focused and on track.

The quality of a person's life is in direct proportion to their commitment to excellence, regardless of their chosen field of endeavor.

—*Vince Lombardi*

CHAPTER 7

Sustain

"Everything, without exception, requires additional energy in order to maintain itself. I knew this in the abstract as the famous second law of thermodynamics, which states that everything is falling apart slowly.... Existence, it seems, is chiefly maintenance." (Kelly, p. 9)

Sustaining our efforts and sticking with the system may end up being the biggest challenge of all. We have moments—maybe many of them—when we have serious doubts about it all, about ourselves, about it being a valid, worthwhile program. But think of it this way: **it's basically just a daily routine.** Routines motivate us to get going in the morning. Routines help us stay focused because they reduce the number of decisions we have to make every day.

Making Decisions Can Be a Very Time-Consuming Ordeal

What do I do today? What do I do now? What do I do with the rest of my life? **With a system, a routine, we've already made all these major decisions.**

We can avoid the drifting, directionless confusion that Daisy feels in the F. Scott Fitzgerald classic *The Great Gatsby:* "'What'll we do with ourselves this afternoon?' cried Daisy, 'and the day after that, and the next thirty years?'"

With our routine system in place, we've already made dozens if not hundreds of decisions about what we want to do today and tomorrow and even the rest of our lives. We're free to start working our system every morning. Nice and orderly. Structured. Grounded. Guided by the work we've already done in producing the system.

Such a basic act of *making a decision* can be paralyzing and stultifying. We hem and haw and stall and debate with ourselves and get nothing done while failing to decide.

We need to turn the *Could I? Would I? Should I?* into *I could! I should! I will!*

Put yourself first. Put yourself, grammatically speaking, in the nominative case. Don't be in the objective case, the object of the action. Be proactive. Be the subject of the action. Step up. Take charge. Make the decision to *nominate* yourself.

Tony Robbins calls decision making "the pathway to power."

> *Everything that happens in your life—both what you're thrilled with and what you're challenged by—began with a decision.* **I believe that it's in your moments of decision that your destiny is shaped.** *The decisions that you're making right now, every day, will shape how you feel today as well as who you're going to become.... (pp. 32-33)*

So now, every day, we just need to **stick to the process. Work the system.** Keep reviewing it all, refreshing our memory about it all, taking it in, being mindful of it, finding connections, creating synaptic associations, so that one letter, one word, one idea triggers a rapid chain of signification.

> *Pursue, keep up with,* **circle round and round your life,** *as a dog does his master's chaise. Do what you love. Know your own bone; gnaw at it, bury it, and gnaw it still.—Henry David Thoreau, from Family Letters*

With the system acting as guard rails, we can let our minds loose, like wild horses on a controlled track (this system of galloping words), racing over all the Ps, then the Es, and so on. In doing so, you'll feel invigorated, fired up—literally, with your synapses firing on a supercharged, self-aware, happy-thoughts rush.

Don't underestimate the vital nature of nurturing your thoughts, letting them run through you at top speed, making their own connections and plans for you. When your system takes on a life of its own, you're exponentially more intelligent. And more intelligence produces better results.

Okay, but Just Waking Up & Getting Going Every Morning Can Be Tough

I know. Trust me, I know. Just getting up out of bed can be challenging. I know it is for me sometimes. The physical issues are one thing: bad back, still tired, sore all over. But the mental challenge can be worse: a mind full of doubts, worries, maybe even depression.

Eliminating as a reason actual clinical depression—for which we should definitely seek the help of medical professionals—I believe that Stephen Pressfield, in his classic little book *The War of Art*, has nailed the source and name of that negative force inside us: **Resistance**. We all struggle to overcome an internal, psychological *resistance* to get up, get to work, or even, in more severe cases, to just to carry-on.

> *I wake up with a gnawing sense of dissatisfaction. Already I feel fear....What I am aware of is* **resistance**. *I feel it in my guts. I afford it the utmost respect, because I know it can defeat me on any given day as easily as the need for a drink can overcome an alcoholic. (Pressfield, p. 65)*

I have sleep apnea and wear a mask that pumps air into my nostrils all night long. The effect is the deepest REM-5 sleep and vivid, life-like dreams you've ever experienced. Every night.

I have the most bizarre dreams imaginable. I'm a haunted house and my many ghosts torment my sleep. But that's another story. When I wake up for the final time—anywhere between 4:45 and 6:45 am—I practically leap out of bed. That's my method, anyway. I don't pause or hesitate for a second. I can't think or my thoughts might stop me from getting up. I wake up, punch the off button on the CPAP machine, rip the mask off my face, and get out of bed fast. I launch myself into the day.

Don't even think about it. Just get up and get going.

Fixes to the Bad Morning Mood: Revert to the System. Work the Plan.

Whether we're tired, slow, low, blue, depressed, in doubt, wanting just to be lazy and do nothing, have the blahs—none of that matters. Shake it off. Be tough. Fight the Resistance.

Return to the Structure

We're a building under construction. We're constructing ourselves. Constructing means "with structure." Brick by brick, floor by floor, one hammer blow and screwdriver turn at a time. Left foot, right foot, left foot, right foot. Hannibal led an army of elephants across the Alps one step at a time.

As I write this, it's 8/12/20. I started this book on 7/20/20 and I have 65 pages already constructed. I've a long way to go, but the framework is in place and the building is taking shape. One thought, one idea, one mantra, one word, one piece at a time.

Structure and routine saves us from the resistance, from having to make decisions. Just dive headfirst into the swimming pool of the system, knowing that the cold water and the depth of the pool are our friends. Ed Coan, who is widely regarded as the greatest powerlifter of all time with more than 71 world records, says, *"I love my routine and when nothing upsets my routine"* (Ferriss, *Tools,* p. 313). And the brilliant author Annie Dillard waxes poetic: *"A schedule defends from chaos and whim. It is a net for catching days"* (Ferriss, *Tools,* p. 375).

Every single morning, no matter what the mood or challenges the day presents, we must do our work. Get our heads screwed on straight by reverting to the system.

It's a struggle, for sure, but we should "honor the struggle," as Burchard frames the structure. *"We must anticipate, welcome, and leverage the struggle....This mindset, more than any other, is at the heart of my work.... **When we learn to see struggle as a necessary, important, and positive part of our journey, then we can find true peace and personal power"*** (p. 270).

Honoring the struggle, we get out of bed and launch back into our system.

The Miracle Morning

In his tremendous little book The Miracle Morning, Hal Elrod makes an air-tight convincing case why getting an early start on your day will transform your life. Make it a daily routine to get up, get going, and never deviate from that habit of early rising. Don't react to the world yet. Put yourself first. Prepare your mind for the day by meditating, prioritizing, and visualizing your plan. His SAVERS system for the first hour of every day is brilliant. S is for silence: keep it quiet, serene, meditative. A is for Affirmations: positive thoughts and reminders of your purpose and plans. V is for visualization: picture what you're all about and about to do and then do it. E is for exercise: get your body engaged and energized. R is for reading: get your mind going. S is for scribe: i.e., write. Work your journal or an article or book (Elrod, pp. 51-93).

Pretty much exactly what I've been saying. Have a system, a plan, a routine, and get started on it every morning, every day.

My Morning Routine

1. Mantras. Start repeating them as we go through our bathroom business. *"Everyday....I'm not just surviving....Rage, rage....I'm growing younger...."* I go through all my favorites to remind my lizard brain that *I'm* in charge. I don't succumb to the bully in me that wants me to cower and retreat back to bed or go watch TV. Nope. It's another glorious day to make progress, be disciplined, have a purpose, work my program, love my system, and grow younger.

2. Avoid distractions. I only look at the phone to check texts and emails. SM, the news, all that stuff is a potentially day-killing distraction. It can all wait or even go entirely without us for the day, or week, or however long we want to stay on our *low-information diet.*

3. Gratitude! Think of all we're grateful for. *"I do gratitude practice every morning, every day....I just know if I do it, I feel better....it's a very effective method to instantly change how you're feeling"* (Turia Pitt, from Ferriss, *Tribe*, p. 168).

4. Water up. Drink LOTS of ice-cold water. Don't skip this tip. Cold water wakes us up—lots of cold water. Gulp, gulp, gulp. Need that liquid oxygen for the brain. Your body's dehydrated from the long night sleeping. The benefits and necessity of drinking water in the morning are legion.

5. Coffee time! This is debatable, of course. But I'm on the pro-coffee side of the argument. (See my full discussion of the pros and cons of coffee in the Eating chapter.)

6. Stretch. I do some spine, leg, and full body stretches. They don't have to be too elaborate or time-consuming. I just primarily work my back to get the spine going and release the magical dogs of the mood and attitude war: endorphins.

   Physical activity, including stretching, increases production of endorphins, the neurotransmitters in the brain that can elevate mood and alleviate pain and depression. Endorphins, small neuropeptides produced by your pituitary gland and hypothalamus, have a chemical composition similar to opiates such as morphine and codeine, which reduce pain. The release of endorphins can produce emotions such as euphoria and enhance the immune system. Hence the term "runner's high," the feeling many runners—and other athletes—obtain from the exercise-induced release of endorphins. (Thomas)

As with so much else I discuss in this book, there are many online resources with videos and pictures to give you some ideas about how to stretch. Here are a couple of simple ones to get you started: https://www.verywell-health.com/stretching-exercises-for-your-back-2696357 and https://www.cbphysicaltherapy.com/stretching-morning-can-change-life/.

7. Meditate. I head to my patio and get my breath and mind under control, calm, at peace, serene.

Once I'm done, I head to my office with my water and coffee and start writing.

You may have another activity for yourself, such as going to your job, obviously, and that's fine. But even if you're not obsessed with writing a book like I am, trying to write in your journal before going to work is a good way of getting started with your day. You can review your goals, updating them by writing specific goals and a schedule for this day, this wonderful opportunity to spend 15 hours or so out of bed, working on you and your life and quest to grow younger.

Getting Through the Day

Sometimes, maybe a lot of times, our energy flags and we have a tough time sustaining our momentum and effort. Those lags and letdowns often happen in transitional moments—the time between doing things, when moving from one task, appointment, place, person, event, or item on our to-do list to another. We've expended a lot of physical or mental energy already. Now we have to deal with the next thing on our agenda, the next phase of the day, the next step in our system. *Always* the *next* task, appointment, event, phase, step, person, place, or thing. That's life. That's our day: moving from one component to the next.

It's precisely in those transitional moments that our energy tends to give out and our resolve diminishes. Burchard notes that *"the most effective way to increase energy is to master transitions."* We should—and must—use such transitional times to restore and amplify our energy. We need to *"release our tension, and set our intention."* We can do so by using conscious breathing and meditation. Actually, while moving from one activity to another is the *perfect* time and opportunity to refocus, reset, be mindful, calm down, and just get our head back in the game and ready for the next activity or part of the day, whatever that is.

In your quick, 1-2 minute mindful meditation, while consciously breathing, just **repeat** *"Release,"* **and focus on feeling the tension flowing out** of your mind, your chest, your neck or wherever it resides. The spend another 1-2 minutes, *"setting your intention"*: **focusing on what's next,** going over "*next* I do this," visualizing yourself doing it and doing it well and happily—or, if not exactly *happily*, since it could be an inherently difficult agenda item—at least *calmly and mindfully*. And then, once you've released your tension and set your intention, you should be ready to go.

Overcoming Obstacles & Excuses: Treat Them as Challenges

Obstacles are opportunities to confront a challenge.

> *...obstacles are those terrible things you see when you take your eyes off the goal. —Henry Ford (from Ferriss, Tools, p. 417)*

> *You can respond to a challenging situation in two ways: you can view it as a challenge or threat and that choice can make all the difference in how it affects you.* (Matthews, p. 171)

Excuses are the *Resistance* in us. Excuses are *us resisting ourselves.* They're self-defeating and self-destructive.

> *...psychoanalytic treatment may in general be conceived of as a reeducation in overcoming internal resistances.—Freud*

> *when man determined to destroy*
> *himself he picked the was*
> *of shall and finding only why*
> *smashed it into because*
> *—e. e. cummings*

Some Common Obstacles and Excuses

- "I'm **too busy** to _____."

Bull. We're not too busy. Consult Covey's Time Management Matrix. We're probably spending too much time on the wrong things. **We need to prioritize. Make better decisions on how to spend our time.** *"I don't believe in 'too busy.' Like I said, busy is a decision. ...You don't find the time to do something; you make the time to do things"* (Debbie Millman, from Ferriss, *Tribe*, p. 24).

- **"I've just got too many problems/obstacles/issues in my way."**

Really? That's life, isn't it? *"**Life is the obstacles**. There is no underlying path. Our role here is to get better at navigating those obstacles"* (Janna Levin, from Ferriss, *Tools*, p. 52).

- **"I can't ignore these other things/my pain/what people say/ how I feel, etc.**

Yes, we *can* ignore them. See Meditation and Mindfulness. We can't make progress, achieve our Goals, realize our success if we can't **ignore what's in our way.** *"Learning to ignore things is one of the great paths to inner peace"* (Robert J. Sawyer, from Ferriss, *Tribe*, p. 91).

- **"It's too painful. It's too hard. It doesn't feel good. It makes me suffer."**

Meditate immediately. You need to get a grip on what's really hurting you: you.

[Before meditation] I didn't understand why there was so much suffering in the world and in my own life, and what could be done about it….The most important thing I realized [from meditation] was that the deep source of my suffering is in the patterns of my own mind. When I want something and it doesn't happen, my mind reacts by generating suffering. Suffering is not an objective condition in the outside world. It is a mental reaction generated by my own mind. (Yuval Noah Harari, from Ferriss, Tools, pp. 558 & 560)

- "I'm **too worried** about things to concentrate on anything else."

Again, see **Meditation and Mindfulness**. We can overcome worry. In the movie *Bridge of Spies,* the Tom Hanks character exasperatedly asks a spy who's under arrest and facing execution, *"Aren't you worried?"* The spy calmly replies: *"Would it help?"* Exactly. **How does worrying help?**

- "I **just can't do it.** It can't be done. I'm not up to it. It won't work."

These doubts are normal but shouldn't be debilitating or dissuade us from pressing on. We just *have* to try. What are we going to do? Never try because we might fail? What kind of weak-willed, self-defeating attitude is that? Turn it around. **Turn those negative thoughts into positive thoughts.** *"Self-doubt can be an ally. This is because it serves as an indicator of aspiration. It reflects love, love of something we dream of doing, and desire, desire to do it"* (Pressfield, p. 39).

It might be hard, but we can do it. *"In this age, which believes that there is a shortcut to everything, the greatest lesson to be learned is that the most difficult way is, in the long run, the easiest."*—Henry Miller

- "I just **wanna quit.** Okay? Sue me. I just wanna quit."

Well, we can't quit. Okay? Sue *me*, lizard brain. I mean, you *can* quit, but I won't let you. It's me against me and I'm going to win, not lose. I'm going to **double down**.

...the next time you catch yourself being average when you feel like quitting, realize that you have only two good choices: *quit or be exceptional. Average is for losers....* *The opposite of quitting is rededication.* The opposite of quitting is an invigorating new strategy designed to break the problem apart. (Godin, The Dip, pp. 44 & 51)

- "There's a lot of **important things going on in the world that I have to pay attention to**. I need to spend time following the news. Then it upsets/angers/sidetracks me."

Tune it out. Ignore it. Stop spending your precious time on news that's outside your Circle of Influence. Revert to a **"low-information diet."** If anything truly important happens, you'll hear about it.

Dealing With Doubts in General

Doubts, self-doubts, doubting it can work or we can do it or it's worth it—they're all products of our lizard brain. Or even the devil, if you will. Don't believe in the devil? How about reframing an evil force in terms of anything acting in opposition to your own best interest—assuming that best interest doesn't hurt anyone else. You're innocently, purely, sincerely just trying to get better. And doubts stand in your way, fighting to defeat you. To me, that's the devil. Or a good word for it, anyway.

Specific Strategies to Deal With Doubts Head-On

1. Breathe.

2. Mindfully meditate, love your mantras, think positive thoughts, take the uptown train.

3. Say *Stop!* I don't wanna hear it. It's my lizard brain screwing with me.

4. Shake it off, slap yourself, "*Snap out of it!*" Take action. Get moving.

5. Associate the negative doubt with a positive memory of the thousand times you've succeeded in doing something that your doubting mind thought you couldn't. Rewire your brain from doubt to "*did it. Been there, done that.*"

6. Write it right out of you. Take a timeout and write in your journal. Work it out on paper. Make the doubts face the music of your thoughts and words. Duke it out in your Gdoc.

7. Acknowledge the doubt. Say, "*Okay, I hear you.*" But then shrug it off. "*I'm moving forward, pressing on, paying no more attention to you. Get out of my way or I'll run you over.*"

8. If you do what you're doubting you can do, what's the worst that can happen? You're not thinking of committing a crime or risking your life, are you? Okay, then. How bad can the consequences of going against your doubts be?

9. Be comfortable being uncomfortable. Get used to it. Practice what John Keats called *Negative Capability*: "*the ability to live with doubts, fears, and uncertainties*" without letting them get to you.

10. Welcome the doubts. They're your friend, an opportunity, a tough opponent that will make you better. Challenges faced are victories earned.

Dealing With Fear in General

Fear is the big one, isn't it? At the root of most of these obstacles and doubts lies fear. We're afraid to commit, to fight forward, to change.

"Everything you want is on the other side of fear."

Either Jack Canfield or George Addair said this first. As an aside, it's interesting how so many inspirational quotes have been attributed to different people. I spent—I almost said wasted—a couple of hours trying to hunt down which of these two men actually said this first. But even the articles that discussed Jack Canfield and George Addair having said this did not convincingly nail it down to either one.

At any rate, quote stealing aside (because one of them is guilty of stealing the other's words!), fear is painful and we naturally want to avoid thoughts and actions that make us afraid. We become cowardly when fearful. For example, if we're tired, we want to avoid the gym. We're afraid of the hard work. When we're tired at night and get hungry, we get weak and eat. *"Fatigue makes cowards of us all,"* said Vince Lombardi.

Fatigue aside, life throws some legitimate bad stuff to be scared of at us. The Chinese Communist Party, criminals, tornados, diseases, unemployment, financial crises, homelessness, assorted heartbreaks, the I-4 corridor, a head-on collision with a tractor trailer. Stuff like that. But this? Following this *PEERLESS* system? There shouldn't be anything too much or too scary to handle here.

Kristen Ulmer, author of *The Art of Fear*, has some remarkably mindful and counter-intuitive insights on the subject of fear:

> *Because my belief is that your relationship with fear is the most important relationship in your life, I now spend at least two minutes a day engaged in what I call fear practice....*

Fear is a sense of discomfort in our bodies. It may show up in obvious ways as fear, stress, or anxiety (which are all pretty much the same thing), or maybe it will feel more like anger or sadness (which can be tied to fear, if fear is in the basement). If it seems like it's in our minds, that's because we're not dealing with it emotionally but rather intellectually, which is never a good idea. I locate the feeling in my body – sometimes it's in my jaw or shoulders, sometimes my forehead. Then, I have a 1 to 2 minute, three-step process:

1. *I spend about 15 to 30 seconds affirming that it's natural to feel this discomfort....*

2. *I spend the next 15 to 30 seconds being curious about what my current relationship is with that discomfort.... I give it my full attention then, and ask what it's been trying to say to me that I haven't acknowledged... I use this time with fear to juice its knowledge like you would juice an orange.*

3. *Then, I spend as long as it takes to feel it. Now, this is important: I don't try to get rid of it. That is not what this is about, because that would be disrespectful to fear. The key is to feel the feeling by spending some time with it, like you would with your dog, friend, or lover. I usually do this for about 30 to 60 seconds. After which, fear, feeling acknowledged and heard, often dissipates.* (Ulmer, from Ferriss, *Tribe*, pp. 552-553)

Wow. **Fear is a living entity inside us.** If we acknowledge it, pay attention to it, juice it, feel it, respect it, spend time with it, and hear it, fear will usually go away. Worth a try, I think.

Sleep: At the Day's End, Get a Good 7-9 Hours

The many benefits of sleep are so obvious and have been proven in literally thousands of studies I don't feel the need to document them here. We all know some people who appear to do fine with just 3-5 hours of sleep per night, but those people are either metabolically blessed or playing with fire—almost literally, since chronic inflammation is caused and exacerbated by too little sleep. You're burning up your body if you don't shut it down nightly for 7-9 hours. Among the many benefits of a good night's sleep are a sharper brain, a better mood, less stress, a stronger immune system, steadier blood sugar, and reduced hunger. Heart disease, high blood pressure, stroke, and diabetes are just a few major health issues proven to be related to poor sleep patterns.

I know it doesn't sound good or even possible to most people, but the ideal sleep time is 9pm to 5am. The world-renowned physiologist and sleep therapist, Dr Nerina Ramlakhan said: *"Going to sleep at 9pm might sound far too early. But the best quality sleep is obtained when your circadian rhythm is at its lowest point, which is between around 9pm and 5am"* (Wilkins).

For what it's worth, that's *my* sleep schedule and it's working great for me.

Supplemental Ss

Sacrifice

The truly successful people make sacrifices. What do you want to give up? How hard do you want to work?

> *The more of yourself that you're willing to sacrifice to your cause, the less perfect you have to be to succeed. You just have to get enough right, enough of the time....do you have the discipline to sacrifice the things you want to do for the thing you know you should do?... The people who win make*

the right sacrifices and the people who lose don't....The willingness to sacrifice immediate gratification for future rewards is highly correlated with the ability to create a better life. (Matthews, p .49-53)

<u>Sounds</u>

Jim Donovan, an old rock drummer turned life coach—with a website full of stuff for sale—has a VERY long promotional video that finally asks us for a mere $39 to learn all the secrets of an ancient soundwave called The Solomon Frequency (SF), which he says can do everything but instantly shave 50 years off our lives. It's completely nuts what he claims that just listening to this one particularly extended note—played by what sounds like a synthesizer—can do for us. I didn't buy his program, but I did find the SF somewhere else on the internet and I won't even share it with you because I found it too painful to listen to. Donovan even tells us to not try driving a car or doing much of anything for 30 minutes after listening to it because it's so powerful. Like I said, nuts. Right? Or not? Maybe there's something to it? He's got dozens of testimonials that listening to SF will change your life.

It doesn't work for me, but it might work for you.

Sounds are pretty personal, subjective, aesthetic sensory experiences. The sound of a voice may arouse or repulse us. Fingernails on chalkboards—kids and even millennials don't know what they missed out on there. Birds chirping, dishwasher humming, crowds at a ballgame, ringing in our ears, iPhone notifications, Amber Alerts, screams, sighs, moans, sirens, waterfalls, agonized crying. Sounds are used for meditation and torture, commands and catcalls, triumphs and disasters.

And music. Ah, sweet music.

I like that old-time rock and roll, hot jazz of Dizzy and Duke and Miles, some country, some swing, some anything. But you might hate what I like and vice versa. And that's fine. My son likes hip hop and rap. Not for me.

Far too minor chord, sullen, and downbeat. I like upbeat. Even the downbeats in jazz are upbeat. And the Blues is majorly beautiful.

I play piano. Have since I was 9. Have written more than 100 songs. Most are pretty bad, but some are pretty good, actually. It's one of the two major disappointments in my life that I didn't succeed in becoming a rock star. Just the thought of it literally makes my heart ache even now, 40 years after my last band broke up.

I played in rock bands from 64-79. Opened for The Who, Allman Brothers, Rascals...

As I write this at 9:24 AM 8/19/20, I can feel those sweet memories and hear the sounds of music in Code 1, the #1 rock venue in Ft. Lauderdale from 64-69. My band played there many times. I had a Farfisa organ and a Wurlitzer electric piano and I rocked. In 68, I bought a Hammond B-3 from Hale's on the corner of US1 and Oakland Park Blvd. I can remember that event vividly. The B-3 is only THE greatest organ ever made. The big dark brown, almost mahogany one with the four sculpted legs? The one you've seen—if you've ever seen any bands—many times. Boy, I miss that beast. It made sounds that purr. Jimmy Smith? The greatest organist ever? That's his instrument.

For the past many years—from my early 30s to my late 60s—I rarely played the piano. Frankly, the disappointment of my professional failure was too painful. I had to tune it all out. Playing the piano only made me profoundly sad and frustrated. But, I'm finally over it. I've recently started playing again and it's been a wonderful, soothing addition to my life. Sad to say, I'm not very good at it now. My left hand shakes a bit, which has me hitting some wrong notes. Not pleasant to listen to. So I almost always play when no one else is home. I'm determined to play my beautiful piano even though I play poorly, because some skills and experiences are worth doing poorly. Even if we're not good at it, even if we lack talent, it's still worth trying and doing at some level. That's the way I feel about my piano playing. The truth is, I was never very good. That's the real reason why I didn't make it as a rock star. I was okay, but compared to my peers, Elton John and Billy Joel, I was pretty bad. Yet, I love playing the piano, it makes me feel good, it gives my life more joy, so it's worth doing, even if I don't do it so well.

Anyway...I could go on about music all day. Might write another book just about music.

The germane point is this: **Listen to your music.** And if you play an instrument, no matter how poorly, play it anyway. Your body, your mind, your heart, your soul—they all *need* music.

In "*10 Health Benefits of Music,*" the Pfizer Medical Team reports that

> *Studies have shown that when you hear music to your liking, the brain actually releases a chemical called dopamine that has positive effects on mood. Music can make us feel strong emotions, such as joy, sadness, or fear—some will agree that it has the power to move us. According to some researchers, music may even have the power to improve our health and well-being,....such as the following positive effects:*

> 1. ***Improves mood.*** *Studies show that listening to music can benefit overall well-being, help regulate emotions, and create happiness and relaxation in everyday life.*

> 2. ***Reduces stress.*** *Listening to 'relaxing' music (generally considered to have slow tempo, low pitch, and no lyrics) has been shown to reduce stress and anxiety in healthy people and in people undergoing medical procedures (e.g., surgery, dental, colonoscopy).*

> 3. ***Lessens anxiety.*** *In studies of people with cancer, listening to music combined with standard care reduced anxiety compared to those who received standard care alone.*

4. *Improves exercise.* Studies suggest that music can enhance aerobic exercise, boost mental and physical stimulation, and increase overall performance.

5. *Improves memory.* Research has shown that the repetitive elements of rhythm and melody help our brains form patterns that enhance memory. In a study of stroke survivors, listening to music helped them experience more verbal memory, less confusion, and better focused attention.

6. *Eases pain.* In studies of patients recovering from surgery, those who listened to music before, during, or after surgery had less pain and more overall satisfaction compared with patients who did not listen to music as part of their care.

7. *Provides comfort.* Music therapy has also been used to help enhance communication, coping, and expression of feelings such as fear, loneliness, and anger in patients who have a serious illness, and who are in end-of-life care.

8. *Improves cognition.* Listening to music can also help people with Alzheimer's recall seemingly lost memories and even help maintain some mental abilities.

9. *Helps children with autism spectrum disorder.* Studies of children with autism spectrum disorder who received music therapy showed improvement in social responses, communication skills, and attention skills.

10. *Soothes premature babies.* Live music and lullabies may impact vital signs, improve feeding behaviors and sucking patterns in premature infants, and may increase prolonged periods of quiet–alert states.

Silence

As much as we love music, the sounds of silence are soothing as well. Silence improves memory, stimulates brain growth, and relieves stress.

> *A 2013 <u>study</u> published in the journal Brain Structure and Function found at least two hours of silence could create new cells in the hippocampus region. Another 2006 <u>study</u> in Heart found silence can release tension in the brain and body in just two minutes. Researchers found it was more relaxing than listening to 'relaxing' music. This was based on changes in blood pressure and blood circulation in the brain. (Borreli)*

In addition, one form of mindfulness meditation is practiced in silence, concentrating on our breathing and paying attention to a mantra or an object, clearing our minds of everything.

> *Silence is the communion of a conscious soul with itself. If the soul attends for a moment to its own infinity, then and there is silence. She is audible to all men, at all times, in all places.—Thoreau's Journals*

Smells

Food. Damn. Have to admit the smell of pizza, spaghetti, fresh bread, and burgers and fries kill me. The temptation rips me up. But I resist.

The *good, beneficial* smells you can fill your homes with are essential oils in a diffuser. Lavender, Peppermint, Rosemary, Sweet Orange. So nice. I have a diffuser on a table behind my desk. Ahhhh. Relaxing and very pleasant. Downright pleasurable.

The benefits of aromatherapy include boosting your immune system, reducing stress, aiding in sleep, killing insects, and purifying the air. Many websites can educate you and sell you oils and diffusers. I like this company, though you should check out several: https://www.rockymountain-oils.com/.

If you want to go deep into essential oils and all their hundreds of uses, the definitive guide is Valerie Ann Worwood's *The Complete Book of Essential Oils and Aromatherapy.*

CHAPTER 8

Singularity & Science

"The term singularity describes the moment when a civilization changes so much that its rules and technologies are incomprehensible to previous generations. Think of it as a point-of-no-return in history."

—*Annalee Newitz*

Sustaining our efforts to follow the system will lead us to a better future for ourselves. We'll be healthier, stronger, happier, and well-positioned to take full advantage of the marvels of medical Science in the Singularity.

Although the term "Singularity" is broad and many-faceted, I'm using it as a shorthand for all the scientific breakthroughs in the not-too-distant future. There's a *singular* purpose to this book: advice for growing younger and living longer. Yet, there's far more to it than that. We really have first to consider the totality of those eventualities.

The Singularity. In total, the word encompasses a vast, imposing and even frightening subject. In the very near future, Artificial Intelligence will far exceed human intelligence, to the point of either being our best friend or our worst enemy.

AI as our worst enemy is the stuff of doomsday science fiction—computers and robotic creatures turning on humans. That could actually happen, according to no less authorities than Elon Musk and Stephen Hawking. Musk said in 2016 that humans may one day be treated like "house pets" by computers unless we get control of AI before it gets control of us.

> *"I am really quite close… to the cutting edge in AI, and it scares the hell out of me," he told his SXSW audience. "It's capable of vastly more than almost anyone knows, and the rate of improvement is exponential."…In 2017, the late physicist Stephen Hawking was similarly forthright when he told an audience in Portugal that AI's impact could be cataclysmic unless its rapid development is strictly and ethically controlled. "Unless we learn how to prepare for, and avoid, the potential risks," he explained, "AI could be the worst event in the history of our civilization." (Thomas)*

Stuart Armstrong at the *Future of Humanity Institute* even predicts that AI poses an "extinction risk" to human civilization. An Oxford University professor, Armstrong believes that

> *we could be opening a Pandora's box.… "If AI went bad, and 95% of humans were killed then the remaining 5% would be extinguished soon after. So despite its uncertainty, it has certain features of very bad risks.… The threat of such a powerful computer brain would include near-term (and near total) unemployment, as replacements for virtually all human workers are quickly developed and replicated, but extends beyond that to genuine threats of widespread anti-human violence." ("Artificial Intelligence Poses an Extinction Risk")*

Mass extinction, humans becoming slaves to machines, a complete blurring and erosion of boundaries between humanity and machines. The list of potentially catastrophic end-time events is long and terrifying.

So why did I choose the Singularity as my last "S" and ultimate goal to reach in the *PEERLESS* system? Precisely *because* the future is so uncertain and potentially wondrous or disastrous—for us individually and collectively. If we can control AI, it will produce ways for us to reverse our aging and live well into our 120s, 130s, or beyond.

I don't know about you, but I want to be there in the future. I want to see the Singularity play out. I see myself as someone who might make a difference, a contribution. Going back to first things, first principles, my MS: I want to protect and support my wife, kids, and grandkids. If the doomsayers are right and the future is a horror show for humanity, I need to be there for my family.

Sounding crazy now, isn't it? If anything can happen, anyone can do it. I can't die and leave my family to fend for themselves. I know it sounds crazier with every sentence. But I didn't dream up these worst-case scenarios myself.

In just one of many such conferences, in 2017

> *a team of experts gathered for Arizona State University's (ASU) 'Envisioning and Addressing Adverse AI Outcomes' to talk about the worst-case scenarios that we could face if AI veers towards becoming a serious threat to humanity. 40 scientists, cyber-security experts, and policy-makers were divided into two teams to hash out the numerous ways AI can cause trouble for the world. The red team were tasked with imagining all the cataclysmic scenarios AI could incite, and the blue team was asked to devise solutions to defend against such attacks. These situations had to be realistic rather than purely hypothetical, anchored in what's possible given our current technology, and what we expect to come from AI over the next few decades. Among the scenarios described were automated cyber attacks (wherein a cyber weapon is intelligent enough to hide itself after an attack and prevent all efforts to destroy it), stock markets being*

manipulated by machines, self-driving technology failing to recognize critical road signs, and AI being used to rig or sway elections. (Javelosa)

As we have recently learned, there already are a lot of forces at work rigging and swaying elections, but *"automated cyber attacks"* sound like the darkest future worlds depicted in numerous sci-fi movies.

So, that's Singularity's downside: The End of Humanity as We Know It.

But let's assume for positivity's sake, that we triumph over AI and it remains under our control and not vice-versa. Let's put aside all the doomsday scenarios and just focus on a hopeful, stable future for humanity. What can we expect?

Singularity's Upside is the Beginning of Humanity's Longer Lifespan

By 2030 or 2035, medical advances will allow us to extend our lives another 40-50 years.

The Premise: Humans *Can* Live Well Into Their 100s

"A growing body of research suggests that aging is an entirely preventable condition and that there may be a variety of ways to treat it, from lifestyle changes to dramatic genetic interventions" ("A new anti-aging therapy").

That's just a mildly conservative quote, a teaser. Here's a stronger dose from Ray Kurzweil, one of the leading authorities on the Singularity:

> *Our health technologies are subject to what [I] call the law of accelerating returns, a doubling of capability every year. This means that the ability to understand, model, simulate, and reprogram the information processes underlying disease*

and aging processes will be 1000 times more powerful in one decade and 1 million times more powerful in two decades. (Transcend, p. XVII)

In other words, scientists and doctors will soon have in AI a superhuman ally in their quest to create and manufacture "cures" to aging.

Because aging doesn't *have* to happen. The eminent Nobel Prize winning physicist, Richard Feynman famously said: *"There is nothing in biology yet found that indicates the inevitability of death."*

Dr. Sinclair, echoes this belief: *"There is no biological law that says we must age. Those who say there is don't know what they're talking about"* (*Lifespan*, p. xxiii). In fact, the thesis of his book and his life's research are astoundingly profound. I shared this quote on the first page, but here it is again:

> *I believe that aging is a disease. I believe it is treatable. I believe we can treat it within our lifetimes. And in doing so, I believe, everything we know about human health will be fundamentally changed.* (Sinclair, p. 81)

If getting old is a disease and it's actually *"treatable,"* as Dr. Sinclair claims, then we can all live a whole lot longer than we've previously imagined.

A Brief History of the Anti-Aging and Reverse Aging Movement

This discussion of and research into the science of longevity and reverse aging has been going on for quite some time—since the early 1990s at least—with most of us in the general public being oblivious to it. Unfortunately, scientists who have been seriously and carefully studying the causes of and potential "cures" for aging have had their efforts undermined by thousands of assorted quacks, charlatans, and cons in the "treatment" and supplement game. Wild promises that some form of meditation or magnet or miracle food or drug would cure whatever ails you and even send you on a course of growing younger have been this age's snake oil. These hucksters have done enormous harm to the legitimate anti-aging community and its reputation, as truly brilliant scientists doing genuinely remarkable work have been lumped together with this motley crew of opportunists selling their miracle potions and plans without a shred of factual evidence that they work. As a result, those who do the actual work of "prolongevity" have to struggle mightily for funding that only comes with a perceived legitimacy of that work.

In 1996, Dr. Michael Fossel published his landmark book *Reversing Human Aging,* the first history of why and how aging occurs. In his latest book, *The Telomerase Revolution,* he makes the case that telomerase is the enzyme that "*holds the key to human aging.*" Along with making that case, he details his friendship and collaboration with numerous iconic and legendary scientists in their quest to prevent and reverse human aging. The stories he tells are fascinating and profound, including how Mike West founded Geron, "*the first biotech corporation aimed directly at preventing and reversing human aging*" (p. 48). He records how Dr. Leonard Hayflick, "*one of the most remarkable scientists in history,*" came up with his famous Hayflick Limit: that cells can divide only a fixed number of times (p. 40-60), proving that "*cells don't age because of the passage of time; cell divisions cause the cell to age....strongly suggest[ing] that aging occurs within cells, not between cells*" (p. 21-22). Furthermore, Dr. Fossel relates how Dr. Cal Harley "*proved that telomere shortening was not only correlated with cell aging, but that it actually caused cell aging...[and that by] Using telomerase, we could turn back the clock, making an old cell young again*" (p. 56-57).

In 2007, Dr. Aubrey de Grey and coauthor Michael Rae published *Ending Aging,* a universally praised and respected guide to the many advances in cellular and molecular biology that could reasonably be expected to lead to significant anti-aging therapics. Based on existing, peer-reviewed research, de Grey coined the term SENS (for "strategies for negligible senescence") to describe his approach to combatting aging. His progress since then has been steady and remarkable, as detailed on his website *The Methuselah Foundation* (http://mfoundation.org).

In 2019, Dr. David Sinclair published *Lifespan*, from which I've already liberally quoted regarding the very real prospects of humans soon being able to live healthy and well into their hundreds. One of his main projects is TAME ("Targeting Aging with Metformin"), a proposed study—waiting for enough funding to move forward—on the diabetes drug Metformin, which shows great potential to do much more than just treat diabetes. If the clinical trial proves its points, the USFDA *"has agreed to consider aging as a treatable condition"* (p. 127). Achieving that goal of approving Metformin to treat aging would be a historic game changer because it would recognize that aging is a disease and the healthcare industry, including insurance companies (Medicare and all others), would have to subsidize its treatment. The "points" TAME aims to prove are what several research studies have already found: *"The beauty of Metformin is that it impacts many diseases.... People taking Metformin were living notably healthier lives—independent, it seemed, of its effect on diabetes.... Metformin mimics aspects of calorie restriction....Metformin reduces the likelihood of dementia, cardiovascular disease, cancer, frailty, and depression, and not by a small amount"* (p. 124-126).

Dr. Fossel, Dr. Sinclair, Dr. de Grey, and many of their colleagues, peers, and teams of scientists—and other teams elsewhere—hope to enhance their traditional research methods with AI technology:

> *...the science is moving fast, faster now than ever before, thanks to the accumulation of many centuries of knowledge, robots that analyze tens of thousands of potential drugs each day, sequencing machines that read millions of genes a day, and computing power that processes trillions of bytes of data at speeds that were unimaginable just a decade ago. Theories on aging, which were slowly chipped away for decades, are now more easily testable and refutable.* (Sinclair, p. 18)

Toward the end of this chapter, I will detail many current clinical studies and trials, including the specific companies, labs, and institutes conducting that research. Before we get there, however, let's discuss and better understand those specific "theories on aging."

So What Exactly Happens to Us As We Age?

Why do our bodies and minds wear out and die? If we can pinpoint the main reasons and causes—and we have—then we can work on the cures—which we are.

> *Aging is not a single process. It consists of a dozen or so processes, each of which leads over time to loss of physical, sensory, and mental capabilities. We [can] dramatically slow down these processes, in many cases stop or even reverse them. In this way, you can stay young until we have even more knowledge to become even younger. (Transcend, p. XVIII)*

The Hallmarks of Aging

In 2013, a team of scientists, led by Carlos Lopez-Otin, published a landmark paper entitled "The Hallmarks of Aging," in which they identified nine symptoms or signs of aging. These hallmarks are not *aging* itself. They are each aspects of aging and shed light individually and collectively upon aging, but it's important to note that aging is a process, not a combination of symptoms, however impressive the list may be.

More importantly, we hope to identify the source of them all, like locating the upstream source of a river that branches into many tributaries. These hallmarks are tributaries and it is likely that their source and our earliest point of intervention is the cellular senescence that occurs when telomeres shorten, leading to DNA unraveling and the resultant alterations in gene expression, which lead to that degeneration of cellular health. A process, not a collection of symptoms.

In an email exchange, I recently had with Dr. Fossel—who has been most generous with his time and tutelage—he makes the following analogy to the Covid-19 virus:

Covid-19 Symptoms:

- *Fevers or chills*

- *Cough, SOB*

- *Fatigue*

- *Head & body aches*

- *Loss of taste or smell*

- *Sore throat*

- *Nasal congestion*

- *Nausea & vomiting*

- *Diarrhea*

But these are not Covid-19 itself. Covid-19 is a dynamic <u>process</u> occurring when the virus enters a human body. We can list symptoms (just as we can list aging biomarkers), but Covid-19 is a disease process, not a set of symptoms. Aging is likewise a process, not a set of biomarkers. (Fossel, 11/20/20 email)

With these distinctions in mind, the 9 hallmarks that Lopez-Otin and colleagues identify and discuss are: genomic instability, telomere attrition, epigenetic alterations, loss of proteostasis, deregulated nutrient sensing, mitochondrial dysfunction, cellular senescence, stem cell exhaustion, and altered intercellular communication.

Let's define each one and then discuss their possible preventions or treatments. The DNA tag 🜨will mark specific research underway by doctors and scientists. (I use this tag very loosely and as a general symbol, since not all of the research involves DNA). The Action tag ≊ will mark specific things we can be doing to help ourselves.

Genomic Instability

A genome is the genetic material, the DNA, of an organism. Genomic instability (aka genetic instability) refers to a high frequency of mutations and damage within the genome of a cell. This condition leads to many cancers, tumorigenesis, and accelerated aging. Its external causes include smoking cigarettes, PCBs, the chemicals in plastics, sodium nitrate that's in most cured meats (especially bacon), UV light, x-rays, gamma rays, and radon in homes (Sinclair, p. 113).

Alcohol can also cause DNA damage:

> *When alcohol is metabolized, acetaldehyde is formed. Acetaldehyde causes a dangerous kind of DNA damage— the interstrand crosslink (ICL)—that sticks together the two strands of the DNA. As a result, it obstructs cell division and protein production. Ultimately, an accumulation of ICL damage may lead to cell death and cancer. ("Scientists")*

Internal causes of DNA damage include DNA replication defects and/or a failure by our bodies' own repair mechanisms. When DNA gets damaged, our bodies engage various mechanisms, including chemical reversal, excision repair, and double-stranded break repair.

Critical to aiding in those repairs is a family of proteins known as sirtuins. Playing a key role in cellular homeostasis—keeping the cell in balance— sirtuins selectively regulate the activity of many key genes responsible for metabolism, inflammation, and cell defense and repair. However, sirtuins can only function in the presence of NAD (nicotinamide adenine dinu-cleotide), a coenzyme found in all living cells that *"boosts the activity of all seven sirtuins.... Without any NAD, we'd be dead in 30 seconds. NAD is a central regulator of many major biological processes, including aging and disease.... NAD acts as fuel for sirtuins"* (Sinclair, p. 134).

🧬 Another protein, newly discovered, exhibits exciting possibilities for repairing damaged DNA:

> *Scientists have developed a technique for repairing damaged DNA. The breakthrough, published this week* in the jour-nal Nature Communications, *could pave the way for new therapies for cancer and neurodegenerative disorders.... researchers have discovered a new protein called TEX264 that can combine with other enzymes to find and destroy toxic proteins that bind to DNA and trigger damage.* (Hays)

🧬 In their continuing research to crack the longevity code, scientists are focusing on engaging our bodies' survival and repair mechanisms:

> *By engaging our bodies' survival mechanisms in the absence of real adversity, will we push our life spans far beyond what we can today?...There will come a time in which signifi-cantly prolonged vitality is indeed only a few pills away.... Drugs that engage the ancient survival mechanisms within us are just one of the many ways that* **scientists, engineers, and entrepreneurs are setting the stage for the most sig-nificant shift in the evolution of our species since forever.** *(Sinclair, p. 144-46)*

🧬 Another potential treatment may be right in our own backyards. Various plants experiencing stress have already produced many health-promot-ing molecules, including metformin from lilacs and quercetin from fruits. *"Plants that are stressed have higher concentrations of xenohormetic molecules that may help us engage our own survival circuits. Ever wonder why organic foods, which are often growing under more stressful conditions, might be better for you?"* (Sinclair, p. 131)

📖 Although there are no surefire ways we can repair our own DNA, we can certainly assist our bodies' own repair mechanisms through <u>autoph-agy.</u> Defined as "self-eating," during autophagy, cells consume their own waste or unused organelles and proteins as a metabolic process. A survival mechanism, autophagy is the way that our bodies protect themselves in response to "good stress" (from <u>exercise and exposure to cold</u>) and nutrient deprivation (from <u>intermittent fasting</u>) by clearing out damaged cells that trigger inflammation.

📖 Trigger autophagy and reduce inflammation through <u>intermittent fast-ing, exercise, and exposure to cold</u> by taking ice baths and cold showers, and swimming in cold lakes and oceans.

📖 Since toxicity, oxidation, and inflammation can all contribute to DNA damage, <u>eat more vegetables and fruits </u>for their antioxidant and anti-in-flammatory qualities.

📖 <u>Eat sirtuin-rich foods,</u> such as blackcurrants, kale, olives, olive oil, pars-ley, capers, onions, and fish (especially salmon and tuna).

📖 Drink green tea.

📖 Take these supplements: Omega-3 Fish Oil, turmeric, and an NAD+ booster, such as NMN or Tru Niagen. Evidence from several studies sug-gests that when activated sirtuins can help repair DNA and support the healing of brain tissue, blood vessels and more.

📖 Reduce "bad stress" through <u>mindful meditation and conscious breathing.</u>

Telomere Attrition

The stretches of DNA at the end of chromosomes, telomeres protect our genes by keeping chromosomes from fraying and clumping. Serving as a biological clock, shortened telomeres are closely associated with aging, heart disease, diabetes, osteoporosis, muscular dystrophy, and cancer.

Acting as caps on the ends of our DNA strands, telomeres are like the plastic tips on the ends of shoelaces. Without them, the shoelaces unravel—just as our DNA unravels when telomeres shorten. When our telomeres get too short, our DNA is unprotected, so that when cells divide, the resulting errors cause cancer and other fatal conditions.

The scientific consensus is that telomeres become shorter mainly from attrition due to aging. Factors that affect this attrition are oxidative damage, inflammation, smoking, poor sleep, stress, obesity, and toxins in the environment and our food.

Preserving shortened telomeres is the job of Telomerase, a protein enzyme, that unfortunately often becomes depleted due to toxins in food and the environment.

Dr. Fossel is one of the world's leading experts on telomeres and their effect on aging. It's worth quoting extensively from his book for us to understand the profound effect of shortened telomeres on aging and how re-lengthening them by activating telomerase could be the key to a longer, healthier life.

> The research now suggests that if we can alter telomere length, we might be able to slow, possibly even, reverse, aging (23)....Cells with telomerase can maintain themselves indefinitely. Cells without telomerase slowly go downhill (28)... the key to intervening in age-related diseases is employing telomerase to re-lengthen telomeres (39)....Using telomerase, we could turn back the clock, making an old cell young

(57)....we know that telomerase activators work to reverse aging and that nothing else does (186)....In every case, without exception, resetting aging has been accomplished by re-lengthening the telomere, thereby resetting the pattern of gene expression. (p. 187)

🧬 *"An enzyme called ATM Kinase normally involved with DNA repair has been suspected for some time to help lengthen telomeres as well, and after the new test was perfected they tested this new enzyme for activity. It was indeed lengthening the telomeres"* ("Resetting").

🧬 A new procedure developed by scientists at the Stanford University School of Medicine utilizes a *"modified type of RNA to quickly and efficiently increase the length of human telomeres....Skin cells with telomeres lengthened by the procedure were able to divide up to 40 more times than untreated cells. The research may point to new ways to treat diseases caused by shortened telomeres"* ("Telomere Extension").

🧬 Researchers at the *Dana-Farber/Boston Children's Cancer and Blood Disorders Center "identified several small molecules that appear to reverse this cellular aging process. Suneet Agarwal, the study's senior investigator, hopes at least one of these compounds will advance toward clinical trials....'We envision these to be a new class of oral medicines that target stem cells throughout the body,' Agarwal says. 'We expect restoring telomeres in stem cells will increase tissue regenerative capacity in the blood, lungs, and other organs affected in DC and other diseases'"* ("Breakthrough").

🧬 Researchers at the *Institute of Molecular Biology (IMB)* and Johannes Gutenberg University Mainz (JGU) have *"discovered that an RNA molecule called TERRA helps to ensure that very short (or broken) telomeres get fixed again....The researchers expect their work to be applicable to humans as well. Their next step will be to look into these processes in human cells and interrogate their implications for ageing and cancer"* ("How Telomeres").

🏋 Exercise. *"Those who exercise more have longer telomeres"* (Sinclair, p. 102).

🏋 Meditation, due to its stress-relieving benefits, *"has been proven to improve the strength and length of telomeres....A 2015 Canadian study linked evidence of longer telomere strands to meditation (when compared to those who did not meditate)"* ("Top 6").

🏋 Maintain a healthy weight. Obesity leads to shorter telomeres.

🏋 Eat foods rich in antioxidants like vitamin C (red peppers, kale), anthocyanins (blueberries) and polyphenols (dark chocolate, cloves, olive oil).

🏋 Take a supplement that reduces inflammation and fights oxidative stress. In particular, N-acetyl-cysteine (NAC) supports the body's production of one of the few and essential internal cellular antioxidants, Glutathione.

🏋 Consider taking TA-65. Its bioenhanced astragalus (*"steroidal molecules extracted from the root of the astragalus plant"* (Fossel, p. 62)) is a clinically-proven telomerase activator. Developed and sold by T. A. Sciences, https://www.tasciences.com/, TA-65 isn't cheap, but its science is backed by more than 20,000 published articles. Dr. Fossel reports that in two studies conducted on people who have taken TA-65, *"there was evidence that telomere lengths were affected in most patients, and in both studies there was evidence of 'rejuvenation'"* (p. 184). Consequently, he conservatively concludes that *"Ta-65 has supporting data and may have health benefits"* (p. 185). For what it's worth, that's good enough for me: I started taking it in October, 2020, and am cautiously optimistic it'll do some good. Worth a try.

🏋 If you want to know more about your own average telomere length, there are direct-to-consumer tests that will give you your ATL, and compare it to the averages of others in your age group. TeloYears is one such company: https://www.teloyears.com/home/.

Epigenetic Alterations

Epigenetics is the instruction manual for assembling our DNA building blocks. In fact, "...*genes are less important than gene* expression," Fossel, p. 13). These epigenetic instructions assure that each cell knows what cell to be—that a kidney cell becomes a kidney cell and a pancreas cell becomes a pancreas cell. As we get older, our cells experience changes to their gene expression that harm their functions, causing our immune system to fail, thus leading to cancer and other diseases. *"Aging is caused by overworked epigenetic signalers responding to cellular insult and damage"* (Sinclair, p. 48).

As usual, inflammation is a major culprit implicated in epigenetic alterations. Because our metabolic rate and epigenetic alterations are closely linked with inflammation, a vicious cycle ensues, leading to continual *"cellular insult and damage."*

Perhaps the best way to fix these alterations is through cellular reprogramming, which resets cells to a developmental state, thus reverting epigenetic changes. Think of a cell as a computer. It's been factory-programmed, contracted a virus, become dysfunctional, and the best approach to fixing the problem is to do a factory reset.

> *Reprogramming allows scientists to completely reverse the effects of aging, at least on a cellular level. In this method, four proteins are added to older cells to reset them to an embryonic-like state, and it is one of the unique examples of procedures that reverse cellular age. By applying insights gained from reprogramming, it might be possible to more profoundly understand and manipulate what happens as we age. ("Resetting the biological clock")*

This reprogramming alters the genes in adult cells by introducing "transcription factors," a family of proteins that is vital for routine cellular functions and response to diseases.

Dr. Sinclair is a major proponent of reprogramming:

> *What if we could reset the aging clock and prevent cells from ever losing their identity and becoming senescent in the first place? Yes, the solution to aging could be cellular reprogramming, a resetting of the landscape—the way, for instance, that jellyfish have been shown to do by using small body fragments to regenerate polyps that spawn a dozen new jellies.... (Sinclair, p. 158)*

☙ *In the area of cellular reprogramming, "there are a rapidly increasing number of approved gene therapy products and hundreds of clinical trials underway" (Sinclair, p. 160).*

☙ In the Sirtuin family of NAD enzymes responsible for genome maintenance, *"SIRT6 exemplifies an epigenetically relevant enzyme whose loss of function reduces longevity and whose gain of function extends longevity in mice....understanding and manipulating the epigenome holds promise for improving age-related pathologies and extending healthy lifespan"* (Lopez-Otin, p. 7).

☙ In cancer research, drugs are in development that can reverse cellular changes and return cells to their pre-cancerous state.

▦ The usual "home remedies" apply: keep inflammation to a minimum by losing weight, reducing stress, and avoiding toxins in food and the environment.

Loss of Proteostasis

Protein homeostasis or 'proteostasis' is the process that maintains the health of cells by preserving the critical three-dimensional structure of their proteins, which are complex molecules that, in turn, regulate almost everything in our bodies. Made up of hundreds of amino acids, proteins are critical for the proper structure and functioning of tissues and organs.

Proteins come in several varieties, according to their functions, including antibodies that help protect the body from bacteria and viruses, and enzymes that carry out the cells' thousands of chemical reactions.

When things go wrong, it's either because there are too many or too few proteins, or they become misshapen or misfolded and fail to do their jobs. Over time, the malfunctioning proteins accumulate which leads to diseases.

🧬 There are many potential approaches in development to address the loss of proteostasis. One is to inject "chaperone" proteins that act as stabilizers. This theory is currently undergoing trials to assess its effectiveness and safety. Another is to give the patient rapamycin or a proteostasis-regulating drug, such as Metformin, that essentially round-up and clear out malfunctioning proteins.

📜 Reducing caloric intake encourages the breakdown of unused or damaged cellular proteins for fuel, which has the beneficial effect of clearing out damaged proteins.

Deregulated Nutrient Sensing

We could be eating all the right foods and providing our body with all its essential nutrients, but if it's not processing those nutrients, all our efforts are in vain. Nutrient sensing is the body's fundamental process of identifying and regulating nutrients, directing them to where they need to go. Our bodies' building-blocks—such as proteins, amino acids, sugars, and lipids—travel along pathways governed by this sensing system, which also controls the cellular processes of growth and cell division.

These four pathways of nutrient-sensing are associated with four key protein groups that influence aging by regulating metabolism: IGF-1, mTOR, sirtuins, and AMPK. Cells evolved these molecular pathways because it's critical to their survival to have an efficient, fast response to deficiencies in nutrient levels. In the presence of growth factors (specific proteins that stimulate growth) and properly sensed and regulated nutrients, cells proliferate. Conversely, when deregulated nutrient sensing occurs, such as in diabetes, obesity, and aging, the body is vulnerable to the onset of various diseases, which triggers a vicious cycle of further deregulation.

Playing a critical role in the maintenance of nutrient sensing, the liver and muscles are the primary hosts for nutrient processing, which involves oxidizing muscle fat, synthesizing protein, and catabolism, the phase of metabolism in which energy is produced by the breakdown of complex molecules, such as starches, proteins and fats, into simpler ones. Aiding in this process are MicroRNAs, which target the genes that encode the proteins and enzymes in the nutrient-sensing pathways (Mico).

🧬 Scientists are studying various rejuvenation strategies.

🧬 Many studies published in scientific journals, including Mico's, conclude that the best approach is caloric restriction through a healthy diet and intermittent fasting.

🏋 Adopt the Mediterranean diet, which is cited more than any other. The usual: fruits and vegetables, low carbs, no sugars, lean proteins, no processed foods, etc.

🏋 Start intermittent fasting.

🏋 Take a daily anti-inflammatory drug, as simple as aspirin.

Mitochondrial Dysfunction

The decaying of mitochondria is a key driver of aging. Our cells' "power plants," the mitochondria are small, energy-producing structures. The several thousand mitochondria in each of our bodies' cells—a total of more than a quadrillion in our bodies—process oxygen and convert nutrients from food into 90% of our bodies' energy. They also sense dangers and threats to cellular integrity, altering cellular metabolism to help protect the cell from further injury. "*When your mitochondria start to slow down and*

*create an excess of free radicals, the result is widespread chronic inflamma-
tion throughout your body"* (Asprey, *Super Human*, p. 10).

Dysfunction usually happens when mitochondria shift from energy production into defense mode. A vicious cycle of reduced energy production and
higher reactive oxygen species (ROS) production results in further damage to the mitochondria. When less energy is produced, fragility increases,
aging accelerates, and diseases ensue, including Alzheimer's, muscular
dystrophy, Lou Gehrig's disease, diabetes, and cancer. Mitochondrial diseases can affect almost any part of the body, including the cells of the brain,
nerves, muscles, kidneys, heart, liver, eyes, ears, and pancreas.

Dysfunction occurs due to another disease or condition, or as a result of a
poor diet, stress, toxins in our food and environment, or an adverse reaction to drugs or infections. It can also be due to reduced levels of NAD+,
a main coenzyme assisting in the production of Adenosine triphosphate
(ATP), an organic compound that provides energy to the cells.

🜲 *"The most vital parts of the mitochondrial DNA could be moved to another
part of the cell – the nucleus – giving it access to better DNA repair mechanisms and keeping it away from the source of reactive oxygen species. This
approach has been demonstrated for some of this vital code. Of particular
note, the study proving that this is possible was funded on our crowdfunding
platform Lifespan.io!"* ("Mitochondrial Dysfunction").

🜲 Clinical trials are underway for numerous other drugs that attack the
dysfunction in a variety of ways.

🜲 Cold therapy. *"Activate the mitochondria...by being a bit cold....Take a
brisk walk on a winter day in just a T-shirt... Exercise in the cold... Leave
a window open overnight... Don't use a heavy blanket while you sleep"*
(Sinclair, p. 110).

🜲 Take an NAD+ supplement such as NMN or Tru Niagen.

⛏ Consider taking Timeline's Mitopure, a clinically proven nutrient that can revitalize mitochondria: https://www.timelinenutrition.com/.

Cellular Senescence

As we age, an ever-increasing number of our cells become senescent: they stop dividing and supporting their tissues. They become zombies, effectively dead but still active, sending out chemical signals to surrounding healthy cells, encouraging them to also become zombies. Chronically inflamed, they stop repairing and start destroying tissue, raising the risk of cancer, osteoarthritis, atherosclerosis, and neurodegenerative diseases, such as Alzheimer's and Parkinson's. Although the body's immune system eliminates some senescent cells, and others destroy themselves through apoptosis, many zombies escape and accumulate throughout the body because they have high levels of pro-survival genes. *"If we can kill off senescent cells, we can keep our tissues much healthier for longer"* (Sinclair, p. 18).

The usual suspects cause senescence: obesity, inflammation, oxidative stress, telomere erosion, metabolic dysfunction, and the inhibition of autophagy. The main treatment is to elevate the levels of Forkhead box proteins (FOXO) that regulate longevity by stimulating autophagy, which promotes cellular turnover and maintenance.

🦠 The good news is that a new class of zombie killing drugs known as senolytics are now in human trials to see if the positive results observed in mice translate to humans.

⛏ More good news is that a lot of the usual measures elevate the body's FOXO proteins to promote autography and lower the oxidative stress and inflammation that lead to zombie cells: caloric restriction, intermittent fasting, high-intensity and cardiovascular exercise, and heat and cold therapy, such as ice baths and saunas.

⛏ Consider these supplements, all of which will help round up zombie cells: Curcumin, Quercetin, Resveratrol, Allicin, and Berberine.

🎬 Drink green tea

🎬 Take Fisetin, a natural senolytic. A joint study by researchers at the Mayo Clinic and the University of Minnesota Medical School published in the journal *EBioMedicine* found that Fisetin removed senescent cells from aged mice, thereby improving their health and lifespan. They also determined that reducing zombie cells by just 30% results in far better health and longevity. Trials are underway to see if this holds up in humans.

Stem Cell Exhaustion

Stem cells are supercells that can change their epigenetic settings, effectively becoming any kind of cell the body needs. They're also multi-talented, able to improve tissue function, replace damaged red and white blood cells, and guard the immune system from weakening. When they lose their ability to divide and become exhausted—literally worn out—the body becomes more susceptible to diseases, anemia, frailty, muscle loss, and weaker bones.

The root cause of many diseases, chronic inflammation is also likely the main cause of the deterioration of stem cells. This "inflammaging," a term coined by Dr. Claudio Franceschi from the University of Bologna in Italy, describes such out-of-control inflammation. Likely caused by a combination of factors, including problems in the gut microbiome and zombie cells, inflammaging is literally deadly to both stem cells and the people who are afflicted with it.

🐍 Since stem cell research is so well-funded, many cell therapies already exist and many more are in clinical trials.

🎬 In 2008, I had stem cell therapy on my left knee. It worked pretty well. My knee functioned a lot better for a few years, but gradually deteriorated again due to arthritis. I was told then—10 years ago—that such gradual "wearing off" of the benefits is normal and not to expect permanent improvement. However, stem cell therapy has come a long way since then.

It beats a knee or hip replacement. So, if the time comes when my knees and hips get really bad, I wouldn't hesitate to try stem cell therapy again.

📖 In the past few months, I've been doing a lot to help my stem cells. The best thing we can do is reduce our chronic inflammation by the many steps we've discussed over and over: minimize stress through conscious breathing and meditation, eat a Mediterranean diet of nutrient-dense foods that contain antioxidants, reduce sugar in our diets, get at least 8 hours of sleep every night, exercise for 30-40 minutes 5-6 days a week, practice heat and cold therapy, and take the supplements already recommended, such as turmeric, fish oil, resveratrol, Vitamin D, and probiotics.

📖 Read more about it in this very good, concise article: "Are You 'Inflammaging'? How to Stop the Inflammation that Speeds Up Aging." 9/10/19.

https://vitalplan.com/blog/are-you-inflammaging-how-to-stop-the-inflammation-that-speeds-up-aging.

Altered Intercellular Communication

As we get older, the system of sending chemical messages or signals through our bodies tends to break down. Due to inflammaging, the immune system is compromised, causing muscles to atrophy, bones to lose density, and tissues to degrade. This hallmark of aging is closely associated with other hallmarks, such as cellular senescence, genomic instability, a loss of proteostasis, deregulated nutrient sensing, and a defective autophagy response. Treating one hallmark, in effect, treats them all to some degree.

🧬 Scientists are investigating parabiosis—the merging of the circulatory systems of two individuals, based on the supposition that parabiosis can dilute harmful signals. An attempt to mimic the effect of parabiosis, during the process of apheresis—in which blood is drawn from a donor and separated into its components, some of which are retained, such as plasma or platelets, and the remainder returned by transfusion to the donor—the pro-aging signaling molecules are removed, and the blood is reintroduced.

🐟 Life Biosciences, a company co-founded by Dr. David Sinclair, is investigating peptides, small proteins that may affect intercellular communication to delay aging and increase lifespans.

🐟 Many senolytics that are already in human clinical trials may prove to be effective.

📣 Do everything we've already discussed to reduce inflammation: caloric restriction, intermittent fasting, high-intensity and cardiovascular exercise, and heat and cold therapy, such as ice baths and saunas.

📣 Since the gut microbiome significantly impacts the immune system and metabolism, we can help our intestinal bacterial ecosystem with better eating and probiotics.

The Drill

By now, we should all know what we need to do. Let's call it "The Drill." We can review "The Drill" by referring to 📣 under the 9 Hallmarks of Aging. But I've fleshed it out and summarized it in Appendix B.

The Big 4 Killers to Ward Off

The 9 Hallmarks all either account for or contribute to all the Big 4 Killers.

> *If you're in your 40s or beyond... There's an 80% chance you're going to die of either heart disease, cerebrovascular disease (stroke), cancer, or neurodegenerative disease (Alzheimer's dementia). So any strategy toward increasing longevity has to be geared toward reducing the risk of those*

diseases as much as is humanly possible. (Ferriss, Tools, p. 67)

We touched on the causes and possible preventions of heart disease, cancer, cerebrovascular disease (stroke), and neurodegenerative disease (Alzheimer's dementia). The primary cause of them all may be gastrointestinal disorders in the gut that we talked about in the Eating chapter.

The 3 Longevity Pathways

Now that we know so much about what ages and kills us, what to do and not do, it's abundantly clear that we need to engage our longevity genes. They

work by employing ancient survival circuits....the hormesis program governed by the survival circuit, the mild kind of adversity that wakes up and mobilizes cellular defenses.... Our ability to control all of these genetic pathways will fundamentally transform medicine in the shape of our everyday life. Indeed, it will change the way we define our species. (Sinclair, p. 103 & 126)

Doing *The Drill* affects the three main longevity pathways: mTOR, AMPK, and Sirtuins.

When they are activated, either by low calorie or low amino acid diet, or by exercise, organisms become healthier, disease resistant, and longer lived. Molecules to tweak these pathways, such as rapamycin, Metformin, Resveratrol, and NAD boosters, can mimic the benefits of a low-calorie diet and exercise and extend the lifespan of diverse organisms. (Sinclair, p. 129)

Pathway #1

Mammalian (or Mechanical) target of rapamycin (mTOR) is a cellular signaling pathway that regulates metabolism, cell growth, and survival by controlling the processes that generate nutrients and energy. A reduction in the activity of mTOR has been proven by vast amounts of research to increase longevity. For example, by reducing its expression in mice, their median lifespan increased by 25%. Since activation of mTOR blocks the process of autophagy, mTOR needs to be blocked to facilitate autophagy.

🧬 Scientists are working on blocking mTOR, with no perfect solution yet. Although rapamycin has conclusively been proven to work, it has some serious side effects, such as infections and a tendency to trigger the onset of diabetes. Metformin is promising but as yet also unproven.

📖 To inhibit the mTOR pathway naturally, do *The Drill*, especially intermittent fasting, caloric restriction, exercise, and cold exposure.

Pathway #2

Adenosine monophosphate-activated protein kinase (AMPK), our energy transformer, functions well when we're young, but as we age its activation decreases, resulting in obesity, diabetes, and accelerated aging. An increase in AMPK activation can result in a 20% increase in lifespan, due to suppressing inflammaging and reducing body-fat stores. AMPK also promotes autophagy, limits hypertension, improves cellular health, and reduces the incidence of Alzheimer's disease.

📖 To activate the AMPK pathway naturally, do *The Drill*, especially intermittent fasting, caloric restriction, exercise, and cold exposure.

📖 Some particular supplements act as caloric restriction mimetics, fooling the body into thinking it's starving and thereby triggering the production of AMPK: Curcumin, Resveratrol, Quercetin, EGCg (green tea), and Pterostilbene.

Pathway #3

Anti-aging molecules, the silent information regulator genes (Sirtuins) regulate cellular homeostasis, metabolism, apoptosis, telomere length, and DNA repair. Sirtuins sense the environment in terms of stressors and available energy, and alter the metabolism accordingly to promote survival. However, sirtuins can only function in the presence of NAD+, which, unfortunately, seems to decline with age invariably.

📖 To activate the Sirtuin pathway naturally, do *The Drill*, especially intermittent fasting, caloric restriction, exercise, and cold exposure.

📖 Take an NAD+ booster such as Resveratrol, TruNiagen, or Basis.

The Scientific Community's War on Aging

Hundreds of thousands of brilliant scientists worldwide are working on many of the aforementioned ways to reverse aging and extend the human lifespan to 150 and beyond. Let's look at what 23 of the major laboratories, institutions, companies, and organizations have to say about their efforts, in their own words (in *italics*), from their own websites.

AgeX

AgeX Therapeutics is focused on the development and commercialization of novel therapeutics targeting human aging. We are building upon the foundation of our proprietary technologies such as PureStem® and induced Tissue Regeneration (iTR™) to develop innovative medicines designed to address some of the largest unsolved problems in aging. Through PureStem® we have the ability to generate pluripotent stem cell-derived young cells of any type for potential application in a range of degenerative diseases of aging with a high unmet medical need. iTR™ is our revolutionary longevity platform aiming to unlock cellular immortality and regenerative capacity to reverse age-related changes in the body.
https://www.agexinc.com/

Alkahest

Alkahest is a clinical stage biopharmaceutical company targeting neurodegenerative and age-related diseases with transformative therapies derived from a deep understanding of the plasma proteome in aging and disease.

Alkahest is focusing on plasma fractions called chronokines that they claim fight off many age-related diseases. When chronokines that were lost due to aging are restored to the bloodstream, inflammation is reduced and many functions, such as cognition and motor function, return to a more youthful state. Alkahest is currently developing multiple therapies based on these plasma fractions. https://www.alkahest.com/

Amazentis

Amazentis is an innovative life science company dedicated to employing breakthrough research and clinical science to bring advanced therapeutic nutrition products to life. Our bodies are an orchestration of trillions of cells working together. As we age, some of these cells slowly lose function, resulting in the decline of our performance. If we can manage our health at a cellular level, we can do more toward maintaining good health overall. With that understanding, Timeline's creators have invested over a decade developing a new class of nutrient that boosts our cells' ability to revitalize their function....Our focus is the development of innovative products designed to meet the health needs of an aging population. Our current work builds on modulating Mitochondrial function. starting with Mitopure™ (a proprietary highly pure Urolithin A). https://www.amazentis.com/

Biophytis

Biophytis is a clinical-stage biotechnology company focused on the development of therapeutics that slow the degenerative processes associated with aging and improve functional outcomes for patients suffering from age-related diseases, with a primary focus on neuromuscular diseases.

Our therapeutic approach is aimed at targeting and activating key biological resilience pathways that can protect against and counteract the effects of the multiple biological and environmental stresses, including inflammatory, oxidative and metabolic stresses that lead to age-related diseases. https://www.biophytis.com/en/

BioViva

BioViva targets biological aging where it begins, at the cellular level. Our mission is to increase your healthspan through genetics—thereby helping you live disease-free longer. BioViva's gene therapy development platform at Rutgers University and our bioinformatics program assist in the development of new therapeutics designed to regenerate muscle, restore telomere length, protect against cardiovascular disease, and ward off the degeneration of aging itself. We work to improve your health simply because you deserve it! https://bioviva-science.com/

The Buck Institute

The first independent biomedical research institute in the world focused solely on aging. Our mission is to end the threat of age-related disease for this and future generations. We believe it is possible for people to enjoy their lives at 95 as much as they do at 25, and to achieve that, we're seeking a more comprehensive understanding of the biology of aging itself. https://www.buckinstitute.org/

Elevian

We develop new medicines to restore regenerative capacity, with the potential to prevent and treat many age-related diseases. Our mission is to help people age, unburdened by the diseases of aging.

It has been known for some time now that there are certain pro-youthful factors present in blood which can improve tissue and organ regeneration by their presence. This is one reason why we heal and recover from injury much faster when we are young compared to when we get older. Various researchers have spent the last decade or so investigating the blood trying to discern what factors are beneficial to health and which ones are harmful. Some researchers have demonstrated that when young blood is transfused to older animals more youthful regeneration is the result. The opposite is also true as young animals given the blood from older ones suffer a reduced regenerative capacity and age faster.

Elevian is engaged in the development of a number of therapies that increase GDF11 and other beneficial factors found in young blood, this aim is to then use these factors to restore lost regenerative capacity in older people to maintain health and prevent age-related diseases. https://www.elevian.com/

Life Biosciences

We're a discovery, development, and commercialization ecosystem committed to extending healthy human lifespan by advancing treatments for age-related diseases. Our company combines extensive drug development experience with discoveries from our scientific teams and the world's pre-eminent research and academic institutions, creating a unique approach to identifying and prioritizing research for pre-clinical and clinical development programs.

Multiple molecular pathways operate collectively to regulate biological aging. Each of our platforms targets indications where disease pathogenesis has a clear relationship to the biology of aging. Our goal is to become the leader in epigenetic reprogramming, chaperone-mediated autophagy and mitochondrial uncoupling, and ultimately the leading company in the biology of aging and longevity space. We believe the combination of our team, science, and business model uniquely positions us to achieve this goal. We will bring multiple transformational solutions to patients, thereby realizing our vision of changing the course of aging and age-related diseases if successful.

Conventional Efforts - Medical research traditionally treats the consequences of aging, not the underlying condition. In short, medicine today is geared toward managing outcomes – i.e. diseases that are the downstream results of aging.

This effort devotes resources to identifying a specific molecular process that underlies a particular pathology (i.e. the science of the causes and effects of diseases). It then attempts to develop therapeutics to reduce dysfunction associated with that specific pathology. Examples of this kind of one-process/one-drug effort include reducing cholesterol in the blood by lowering its synthesis using statin drugs, or blocking enzymes that regulate blood pressure with ACE inhibitors.

It is widely understood that many patients treated to date with one-process/one-drug approaches fail to respond adequately. We believe the primary reason for this failure is that current methods merely target the downstream effects of aging. The diseases are being managed rather than addressing the root causes of these disorders.

*A New Approach - Our research pursues an exciting and revolutionary alternative: targeting the pathology and underlying biology of aging itself. Therapies derived from this kind of effort have the potential to treat multiple diseases simultaneously. Our unique structure leverages synergies between platforms and related intellectual property.*https://www.lifebiosciences.com/our-science

Lifespan.io

Crowdsourcing the cure for aging. Our mission is to promote the advancement of biomedical technologies which will increase healthy human lifespan. Thanks to the support of the Lifespan Heroes and as part of our commitment to bringing you the latest news in longevity research, we have created the rejuvenation roadmap. This curated database aims to compile the most promising therapies and technologies in development and chart their progress in one easy to read format. We have divided the projects into their corresponding aging hallmarks for ease of reference and clicking on each icon will take you to some more detailed information about each project. The database will be updated on a regular basis ensuring you have the most up to date overview of the rejuvenation biotechnology field. https://www.lifespan.io

Longeveron

Longeveron is a life-sciences company developing biological solutions for aging and aging-associated diseases. We believe regenerative medicine, through cell-based therapy, is a promising new approach to treating these conditions. Participating in FDA-evaluated clinical trials, we are currently testing our cell-based therapy product for a diagnosable ailment called Aging Frailty, a growing condition impacting approximately 50 million Americans over the age of 60. http://longeveron.com/

Methusaleh Foundation

We incubate and sponsor mission-relevant ventures, fund research, and support projects and prizes to accelerate break-throughs in longevity. Our mission-first culture is pursuing six core strategies to make 90 the new 50 by 2030. https://www.mfoundation.org

Oisin Biotechnologies

Oisín Biotechnologies ground-breaking research and technology is demonstrating that the solution to mitigating the effects of age-related diseases is to address the damage created by the aging process itself.

When cells detect that they have been irreversibly damaged, they enter a non-dividing condition known as cell-cycle arrest, or senescence. It's believed this occurs to prevent cells from going rogue and turning cancerous. Ideally, they should die by the process known as apoptosis, but as we age, more and more frequently they don't. They become zombie cells – unable to kill themselves or resume normal function.

Senescent cells secrete molecules that cause inflammation in an effort to attract immune cells that would usually clear them. But for reasons that are not fully known, as we age, persistently senescent cells accumulate, leading to a vast number of age-related diseases.

Oisín is developing a highly precise, patent-pending, DNA-targeted intervention to clear these cells. As a recent study has shown, clearing senescent cells both reduces negative effects of aging pathologies and also extends median lifespan and survival. https://www.oisinbio.com

ResTORbio

Grounded in biology and informed by a large body of scientific research, our mission is to develop innovative medicines that target the biology of aging to prevent or treat aging-related diseases.

Ongoing research is continually expanding our understanding of the biochemical pathways that regulate aging. These learnings inspired our focus to study the biology of aging in order to develop medicines to prevent or treat aging-related diseases and potentially compress or shorten the time of morbidity while lengthening healthspan – the time we are healthy, active, and disease-free. https://www.restorbio.com/

Revel

REVEL IS COMMERCIALIZING THERAPEUTIC DESIGNER ENZYMES TO DEGRADE THE MOLECULAR DAMAGE THAT ACCUMULATES WITH AGING.

We are addressing one of the hallmarks of aging, and are strategically positioned to develop therapeutics for multiple diseases of aging including osteoarthritis, kidney disease, cardiovascular disease, skin aging, and complications of diabetes. https://www.revelpharmaceuticals.com

Salk

One thing's for certain: we all get older. But the biology of aging is still largely a mystery. As for getting sick as we age—we think that might be optional. At Salk, we are deciphering the molecular and cellular causes of aging, and searching for ways to stave off Alzheimer's disease, diabetes, cancer, cardiovascular disease and other age-related ailments. We're studying how the body heals itself, and we're working on stem-cell technologies that may one day be used to replace organs damaged by injury and disease. They say aging isn't for the timid, but we think bold science could help people stay healthy as they age. https://www.salk.edu/science/research/aging-and-regenerative-medicine/

Scripps Research

You are only as old as your biology says you are. At Scripps Research, we identify the fundamental causes of biological aging at the molecular and cellular level with an eye to fending off age-related diseases that undermine our health as we get older. Aging is central to the onset of many disorders—from cancer to heart disease to Alzheimer's—and we now have the ability to decipher the roles of genetics and lifestyle in the aging process. As we better understand this process, we develop therapeutics to prevent and treat age-related diseases. The ultimate goal is to extend human healthspan—lengthening the period over a lifetime during which a person stays healthy and active. https://www.scripps.edu/science-and-medicine/disease-areas-and-medicines/aging-and-healthspan/

Senisca

Senisca is a biotech spinout company from the University of Exeter, founded in 2020 and dedicated to the development of new approaches to reverse cellular senescence (senotherapeutics).

Our founders are world leaders in molecular and cellular biology and have patent-protected an innovation for the reversal of cellular senescence. This innovation works by restoring the ability of cells to 'fine tune' the expression of their genes to rejuvenate aged cells.

At SENISCA, we are using this knowledge, concerning how and why cells become senescent, to develop a new generation of oligonucleotide-based interventions, to turn back the ageing clock in old cells and to target the diseases and aesthetic signs of ageing. https://www.senisca.com/

Sens Research Foundation

SENS Research Foundation works to develop, promote, and ensure widespread access to therapies that cure and prevent the diseases and disabilities of aging by comprehensively repairing the damage that builds up in our bodies over time. We are redefining the way the world researches and treats age-related ill health, while inspiring the next generation of biomedical scientists.

Many things go wrong with aging bodies, but at the root of them all is the burden of decades of unrepaired damage to the cellular and molecular structures that make up the functional units of our tissues. As each essential microscopic structure fails, tissue function becomes progressively compromised – imperceptibly at first, but ending in the slide into the diseases and disabilities of aging.

SENS Research Foundation's strategy to prevent and reverse age-related ill-health is to apply the principles of regenerative medicine to repair the damage of aging at the level where it occurs. https://www.sens.org/

Sierra Sciences

Aging is a complex and difficult topic that has been the center of attention of many scientists for centuries. That's also what Bill Andrews, Ph.D., the founder of Sierra Sciences, has made his challenge to solve. Aging isn't an accident. We age because our telomeres get shorter and our cells age. Every time our cells divide, our telomeres get shorter and our cells age. Aging is also the cause of a lot of diseases. Research suggests that control of the telomere length has the potential to treat many diseases linked to aging. This is what SIERRA SCIENCES group of scientists led by Dr Andrews has been working on for the last two decades and is close to finding cures that change the way we live our life forever. Human aging can be controlled and stopped. Aging is a disease and it can be cured. https://www.sierrasci.com/

The Sinclair Lab

The Sinclair lab is driven by the belief that humanity can do better and that everyone has the right to the best medical care and maximum lifespan, no matter their gender, social status, or age. Work by our lab and others has shown that the pace of aging is not inexorable or predetermined, but rather can be slowed and even reversed by a variety of approaches. These include activating the body's defenses against aging, deleting senescent cells, and reprogramming cells in vivo. In doing so, we can protect the body against and treat both rare and common diseases including mitochondrial diseases, type 2 diabetes, Alzheimer's disease, cardiovascular disease, and cancer.

Our work has led us to the conclusion that the loss of epigenetic information is likely the root cause of aging. By analogy, if DNA is the digital information on a compact disc, then aging is due to scratches. We are searching for the polish. Our work has led us to identify reprogramming factors that we believe will enable us to reset a cell's epigenetic status and reverse its age. We have developed human-compatible viral vectors to deliver the reprogramming genes to specific tissues or the entire body, thereby causing cells to act younger and wounds to heal faster. Our current focus is on nerve regeneration and the reversal of other symptoms of aging. We see treatments being possible for companion animals and humans to dramatically improve their health and lifespan. https://genetics.med.harvard.edu/sinclair/

TA Sciences

TA Sciences is dedicated exclusively to creating research-based, clinically tested wellness products that help address telomere shortening through the science of Telomerase Activation. https:// www.tasciences.com/

Telocyte

Our mission is not to help anyone "live with Alzheimer's", but to ensure that all of us can live without Alzheimer's. Our mission is to cure Alzheimer's, plain and simple. We intend to save the lives, the minds, and the presence of those who have Alzheimer's now and to prevent anyone from getting Alzheimer's in the future. We are committed to a cure, not to finding a symptomatic treatment, nor to finding a way to merely delay Alzheimer's by a few weeks or months. We are committed to reversing the disease process and to giving patients a return of lost function. We are committed to finding out just how much we can offer our patients. https:// www.telocyte.com/

Turn Bio

The nine well-accepted hallmarks of aging illustrate that aging is a multi-dimensional process. To make real progress, we are addressing all the causes down to the root of the problem. Our platform has demonstrated a youthful reversion of eight of the nine hallmarks of aging. Reversion of the ninth is being currently being developed. https://www.turn.bio/

Unity Biotechnology

Our mission is to extend human healthspan, the period in one's life unburdened by the diseases of aging. Working at the frontier of biotechnology and medicine, UNITY's goal is to halt, slow

or reverse age-related diseases, while restoring human health.
https://unitybiotechnology.com

Live Long Into the 22nd Century

It's not even a matter *if* humans can live until 150 or 180 (as Dave Asprey vows to), but only which of us have the will and determination to position ourselves to do so. Other creatures on earth already live long lives, so why can't humans? Greenland sharks live until they're 150 years old and one individual may have lived more than 500 years. One bowhead whale lived to 211 years old (Sinclair p. 55).

The singularity is real. When artificial intelligence catches up with the miraculous genius of our world's existing scientific community, rapid and profound progress will be made. AI has

> the potential to put every anti-aging research project on the fast track. There is so much information on aging research, that it is impossible for one person, or even a thousand, to absorb a fraction of what is currently available and continually growing every day. Up until now, we have not had the capability to discern or draw viable conclusions from this raw data that could then be used to benefit humanity. The path to increased human longevity goes faster with AI assisting human scientists. ("Curing Aging")

By following this *PEERLESS* system, I'll be alive and well 15-20 years from now when the reverse aging breakthroughs will be mine for the asking. Then I'll start growing younger every month. In 2100, I'll be 150 and we'll take it from there.

Come join me in our quest to reach the 22nd century! What have you got to lose?

Bibliography

Allen, David. *Getting Things Done.* Penguin Books: New York, 2001.

Alonso-Pedrero, Lucia, Ana Ojeda-Rodríguez, Miguel A Martínez-González, Guillermo Zalba, Maira Bes-Rastrollo, and Amelia Marti. "Ultra Processed Food Consumption and the Risk of Short Telomeres in an Elderly Population of the Seguimiento Universidad de Navarra (SUN) Project." *The American Journal of Clinical Nutrition,* 111 no. 6. (June 2020): 1259–66. https://doi.org/10.1093/ajcn/nqaa075.

Araki, Kadya. "Why All Humans Need to Eat Meat for Health." *Breaking Muscle* (n.d.). https://breakingmuscle.com/healthy-eating/why-all-humans-need-to-eat-meat-for-health.

Asprey, Dave. *Game Changers.* New York: Harper Wave, 2018.

—. *Super Human.* New York: Harper Wave, 2019.

Berman, Robby. "Ultra-processed Foods May Accelerate Biological Aging." *Medical News Today.* September 12, 2020. https://www.medicalnewstoday.com/articles/ultra-processed-foods-may-accelerate-biological-aging?.

Binstock, Robert H. "Anti-Aging Medicine: The History: Anti-Aging Medicine and Research: A Realm of Conflict and Profound Societal Implications." *The Journals of Gerontology: Series A,* 59 no. 6. (June 2004): B523–B533. https://doi.org/10.1093/gerona/59.6.B523.

Boominathan, Amutha, Shon Vanhoozer, Nathan Basisty, Kathleen Powers, Alexandra L. Crampton, Xiaobin Wang, Natalie Friedricks, Birgit Schilling, Martin D. Brand, and Matthew S. O'Connor. "Stable Nuclear Expression of ATP8 and ATP6 Genes Rescues a mtDNA Complex V Null Mutant." *Nucleic Acids Research,* 44 no. 19, (2016): 9342-57. https://doi.org/10.1093/nar/gkw756.

Borreli, Lizette. "5 Health Benefits Of Being Silent For Your Mind And

Body." *Medical Daily*. September 2, 2016. https://www.medicaldaily. com/5-health-benefits-being-silent-your-mind-and-body-396934.

Burchard, Brendon. *High Performance Habits*. New York: Hay House, 2017.

Cameron, Julia. "Morning Pages," *The Artist's Way*. April 19, 2017. https:// juliacameronlive.com/2017/04/19/morning-pages-10/.

Castle, Alan. "Can Reading Help My Brain Grow and Prevent Dementia?" (blog). *PsychologyToday.com*, April 11, 2018. https://www. psychologytoday.com/us/blog/metacognition-and-the-mind/201804/ can-reading-help-my-brain-grow-and-prevent-dementia.

Childre, Doc and Howard Martin. *The Heartmath Solution*. New York: Harper One, 2000.

Collins, Cathy. "9 Reasons Why Eating Meat Is Good For Health." *Authority Health*. February 17, 2020. https://www.authorityhealthmag. com/eating-meat-is-good-for-health/.

Conger, Krista. "Telomere extension turns back aging clock in cultured human cells, study finds." *News Center* (blog). *Stanford Medicine*. January 22, 2015. https://med.stanford.edu/news/all-news/2015/01/telomere-ex- tension-turns-back-aging-clock-in-cultured-cells.html.

Covey, Stephen. *The 7 Habits of Highly Effective People*. New York: Simon & Schuster, 1990.

Davis, William. *Undoctored*. New York: Rodale, 2017.

De Grey, Aubrey and Michael Rae. *Ending Aging*. New York: St. Martin's Griffin, 2007.

Divine, Mark. *Unbeatable Mind*. Self-Published, 2015.

Elrod, Hal. *The Miracle Morning*. Hal Elrod International, Inc., 2018.

Ferriss, Timothy. *The 4-Hour Workweek*. New York: Crown

Publishing, 2007.

—. *The 4-Hour Body*. Read by Zach McLarty. New York: Random House Audio; Abridged edition, 2010.

—. *Tools of Titans*. New York: Houghton Mifflin Harcourt, 2016.

—. *Tribe of Mentors*. New York: Houghton Mifflin Harcourt, 2017.

Filsinger, Gabriel. "Resetting the biological clock." *SITN: Science in the news* (blog). Harvard University: The Graduate School of Arts and Sciences. September 2, 2016. 9/16. http://sitn.hms.harvard.edu/flash/2016/resetting-aging-clock-science-age-reversal/.

Fossel, Michael. *Reversing Human Aging*. Quill, 1997.

—. *The Telomerase Revolution*. Dallas, TX: BenBella Books, Inc., 2015.

Gent, Edd. "A New Anti-Aging Therapy Is Starting Its First Human Trial—and It Costs $1 Million." *Singularity Hub*. December 16,2019. https://singularityhub.com/2019/12/16/a-new-anti-aging-therapy-is-starting-its-first-human-trial-and-it-costs-1-million/.

Godin, Seth. *The Dip*. New York: Portfolio, 2007.

—. *Poke the Box*. USA: Do You Zoom, Inc: 2011.

Gundry, Stephen. *The Longevity Paradox*. New York: Harper Wave, 2019.

Hanh, Thich Nhat. *Peace Is Every Step*. New York: Bantam Books, 1991.

Hanson, Rick. *Buddha's Brain*. Oakland, Ca: New Harbinger Publications, 2009.

—. *Resilient*. New York: Harmony Books, 2018.

Harvard Health Publishing. "The Dangers of Sitting." *Healthbeat* (blog). Harvard Medical School. May 2019. https://www.health.harvard.edu/pain/the-dangers-of-sitting.

—."Reading Books May Add Years to Your Life." *Harvard Women's Health Watch* (blog). *Harvard Medical School*. October 2016. https://www.health.harvard.edu/healthy-aging/reading-books-may-add-years-to-your-life.

Hays, Brooke. "Scientists Find Toolkit to Aid Repair of
Damaged DNA." *Science News* (blog). *UPI*. March 9,
2020. https://www.upi.com/Science_News/2020/03/09/
Scientists-find-toolkit-to-aid-repair-of-damaged-DNA/3751583765543/.

Hensrud, Donald M.D. "Does Coffee Offer Health Benefits?"
Healthy Lifestyle: Nutrition and Healthy Eating (blog). *Mayo Clinic*.
February 6, 2020. https://www.mayoclinic.org/healthy-lifestyle/
nutrition-and-healthy-eating/expert-answers/coffee-and-health/
faq-20058339.

Hubrecht Institute. "Scientists discover new repair mechanism
for repairing alcohol-induced DNA damage." *ScienceDaily* (blog).
ScienceDaily, March 4, 2020. https://www.sciencedaily.com/
releases/2020/03/200304140749.htm.

Huffington Post UK. "Artificial Intelligence Poses 'Extinction Risk' To
Humanity Says Oxford University's Stuart Armstrong," December 03,
2014. https://www.huffingtonpost.co.uk/2014/03/12/extinction-artifi-
cial-intelligence-oxford-stuart-armstrong_n_4947082.html.

Javelos, June. "What Would an "AI Doomsday" Actually
Look Like?" *Futurism.com*. March 6, 2017. https://futurism.
com/3-ai-experts-weigh-in-on-possible-end-of-the-world-scenarios.

Johannes Gutenberg Universitaet Mainz. "How telomeres Protect Cells
From Premature Senescence: Researchers Found an RNA Species
Identifying Critically Short Telomeres; publication in Cell." *ScienceDaily*
(blog). *ScienceDaily.com*, June 30, 2017. https://www.sciencedaily.com/
releases/2017/06/170630105013.htm.

Kelly, Kevin. *The Inevitable*. New York: Penguin, 2016.

Kurzweil, Ray. *The Singularity Is Near: When Humans Transcend Biology*.
Penguin Books, 2006.

Kurzweil, Ray and Terry Grossman. *Transcend*. New York: Rodale, 2009.

Lemov, D. *Teach Like a Champion: 49 Techniques That Put Students on the Path to College*. San Francisco, CA: Jossey-Bass, 2010.

Licalzi, Diana. "Science-Backed Habits to Live Past 100." *Inside Tracker* (blog). October 27, 2020. https://blog.insidetracker.com/plan-live-past-100-centenarians.

Lifespan.io. "Mitochondrial Dysfunction." (blog). *Lifespan.io. (n.d.)*. https://www.lifespan.io/mitochondrial-dysfunction/.

Lopez-Otin, Carlos, Maria A. Blasco, Linda Partridge, Mauel Serrtano, and Guido Kroemet. "The Hallmarks of Aging." *Cell*, 153 no. 6 (June 06, 2013): 1194-1217. https://doi.org/10.1016/j.cell.2013.05.039.

Loria, Joe. "Here's Why the USDA Refuses to Label Eggs Nutritious, Healthy, or Good for You." (blog). *Mercy for Animals.com*. May 4, 2017. https://mercyforanimals.org/heres-why-the-usda-refuses-to-label-eggs.

Maltz, Maxwell. *Psycho-Cybernetics*. New York: TarcherPerigee, 1960.

Matthews, Michael. *The Little Black Book of Workout Motivation*. New York: Oculus, 2018.

Maximum Life Foundation. "Curing Aging." (n.d.) https://maxlife.org/curing-aging/.

Mico, Victor, Laura Berniches, Javier Tapia-Belloso, and Lidia Daimiel Ruiz. "NutrimiRAging: Micromanaging Nutrient Sensing Pathways through Nutrition to Promote Healthy Aging." *International Journal of Molecular Sciences,* 18 no. 5 (April 2017): 915. https://doi.org/10.3390/ijms18050915.

Natural Health Sherpa (blog). "The Benefits of Drinking Water in the Morning." September 22, 2015. https://www.naturalhealthsherpa.com/the-benefits-of-drinking-water-in-the-morning.

NDTV. "Sedentary Lifestyle Is More Harmful Than You
　　Think: Here's How." *HealthDoctor* (blog). *NDTV.com*.
　　Updated: June 26, 2020. https://www.ndtv.com/health/
　　sedentary-lifestyle-is-more-harmful-than-you-think-heres-how-2252885.

Organixx.com. "Top 6 Ways to Reverse Aging Naturally." (blog).
　　Organixx.com. August 3, 2020. Organixx.com. https://organixx.com/
　　reverse-aging/.

Perlmutter, David and Alberto Villoldo. *Power Up Your Brain*." New York
　　City: Hay House, 2011.

Persson, Charlotte Price. "The Pros and Cons of Coffee." (blog).
　　ScienceNordic, January 7, 2014. https://sciencenordic.com/
　　cancer-denmark-diseases/report-the-pros-and-cons-of-coffee/1395170.

Peters, Jeanne. "The Food Rx to Reverse Aging." *Empowered Aging*, Ed.
　　Sharkie Zartman. Hermosa Beach, CA: Spoilers Press, 2018.

Pfizer Medical Team. "Ten Health Benefits of Music." *Healthy Living*
　　(blog). *Get Healthy Stay Healthy*. August 30, 2017. https://www.geth-
　　ealthystayhealthy.com/articles/10-health-benefits-of-music.

Pressfield, Stephen. *The War of Art*. New York: Black Irish
　　Entertainment, 2002.

Radiological Society of North America. "Reading, Writing and Playing
　　Games May Help Aging Brains Stay Healthy." *ScienceDaily* (blog).
　　ScienceDaily.com, November 25, 2012. https://www.sciencedaily.com/
　　releases/2012/11/121125103947.htm.

Rawls, Bill. "Are You "Inflammagin? How to Stop the Inflammation
　　that Speeds Up Aging." (blog). *Vital Plan*. September 10, 2019. https://
　　vitalplan.com/blog/are-you-inflammaging-how-to-stop-the-inflamma-
　　tion-that-speeds-up-aging.

Robbins, Anthony. *Awaken the Giant Within.* New York: Simon and
　　Schuster, 1991.

Rush University Medical Center. "Daily Leafy Greens May Slow Cognitive
　　Decline." *Rush Stories* (blog). *Rush.edu.* December 20, 2017. https://www.
　　rush.edu/news/daily-leafy-greens-may-slow-cognitive-decline.

Sanchez-Carrido, Julia and Avinash R. Shenoy. "Regulation and repurpos
　　ing of nutrient sensing and autophagy in innate immunity." *Autophagy,*
　　(2020). https://doi.org/10.1080/15548627.2020.1783119.

Satrazemis, Emmie. "Is Dairy Bad for You? The Science Behind It." (blog).
　　Trifecta Nutrition. April 17, 2018. https://www.trifectanutrition.com/blog/
　　is-dairy-bad-for-you-the-science-behind-it.

Schwingshackl, Lukas, Carolina Schwedhelm, Georg Hoffmann, Sven
　　Knüppel, Anne Laure Preterre, Khalid Iqbal, Angela Bechthold, Stefaan
　　De Henauw, Nathalie Michels, et al. "Food Groups and Risk of Colorectal
　　Cancer." International Journal of Cancer, 142 no. 9. December 6, 2017.
　　https://doi.org/10.1002/ijc.31198.

Shojai, Pedram. *The Urban Monk.* New York: Rodale, 2016.

Sinclair, David A. *Lifespan: Why We Age and Why We Don't Have To.* New
　　York: Atria Books, 2019.

Teicholz, Nina. *The Big Fat Surprise: Why Butter, Meat & Cheese Belong in
　　a Healthy Diet.* New York: Simon & Schuster, 2014.

The Harvard Gazette, Health & Medicine. "Breakthrough
　　to Halt Premature Aging of Cells." April 22, 2020.
　　https://news.harvard.edu/gazette/story/2020/04/
　　study-identifies-potential-drug-treatments-for-telomere-diseases/.

The Longevity Reporter (blog). "Resetting The Clock: New Enzyme
　　Found To Repair Telomeres." 11/14/15 http://
　　longevityreporter.org/blog/2015/11/13/

repairing-the-clock-another-new-enzyme-found-to-lengthen-telomeres (site discontinued).

The Underground Health Reporter. Thomas, Jim. "Does Stretching Release Endorphines?" (blog). *AZ Central*. https://healthyliving.azcentral.com/stretching-release-endorphins-6612.html.

Thomas, Mike. "Six Dangerous Risks of Artificial Intelligence." (blog). *Builtin.com*. January 14, 2019. https://builtin.com/artificial-intelligence/risks-of-artificial-intelligence.

Troncale, Joseph. "Your Lizard Brain," (blog). *Psychology Today*. April 22, 2014. https://www.psychologytoday.com/us/blog/where-addiction-meets-your-brain/201404/your-lizard-brain.

Williams, Mark and Danny Penman. *Mindfulness*. New York: Rodale, 2011.

Willink, Jocko and Leif Babin. Extreme Ownership. New York: St. Martin's Press, 2015.

Young, Shinzen. "The Power of Gone." *The Buddhist Review Tricycle*. (Fall 2012). https://tricycle.org/magazine/power-gone/.

Yousefzadeh, Matthew J., Yi Zhu, Sara J. McGowan, Luise Angelini, Heike Fuhrmann-Stroissnigg, Ming Xu, Yuan Yuan Ling, Kendra I. Melos, et al. "Fisetin Is a Senotherapeutic That Extends Health and Lifespan." *Journal EbioMedicine*, 36 (October 2018): 18-28. https://www.ebiomedicine.com/article/S2352-3964(18)30373-6/fulltext.

APPENDIX A

Bones of Contention

As I've noted throughout the book, many areas and topics are the subjects of mild to severe disagreement among the experts. If you want to write a scholarly paper for publication—which could be done for all the following topics—simply state the opposing viewpoints and then stake your claim somewhere in the middle, in a compromise position. It's the Hegelian Dialectic approach: thesis, antithesis, synthesis. Insert yourself in the synthetic realm and you've authorized yourself, made yourself an instant authority by the very act of writing it down and becoming an author. Throughout this *PEERLESS* system, I've encouraged us to produce ourselves, make of ourselves a production, and *will* a new and better self into existence through the sheer force of relentlessly practicing our daily routine habits. Our writing can do that for us. I encourage you to try your hand at it. This long list is our chance—each of us—to take a stand, make a decision, and choose for ourselves which side, which approach is right for us. Of course, do your own due diligence, your own homework, take extreme ownership, always keep learning, and never close that door of consciousness, your mind.

> *If the doors of perception were cleansed every thing would*
> *appear to man as it is, Infinite. For man has closed himself*

up, till he sees all things thro' narrow chinks of his cavern.—
William Blake, *The Marriage of Heaven and Hell*

Aging

Just what, exactly, is it? The vast majority of people—even doctors and scientists—believe that it is natural and inevitable. We've had a look in this book at a few of those who believe it is neither natural nor inevitable. We've discussed the symptoms and causes, the likely process, source, and earliest point of intervention. We've suggested and even insisted that aging is a disease that can and will be treated. Thousands of studies in a variety of areas have been recorded and summarized in millions of words. An entire anti-aging industry has grown and is flourishing, comprised of close to a million brilliant people dedicated to solving the case and helping us live until 150, 180, 200 years or more. Their faith and determination, grit and guts are driving us toward that goal. It's a fascinating and fabulous journey. I'm on board. Can't really think of much better to do at the age of 70 than try my best to live another 80 years or so. The main reason to do so? Our families need us. Heck, the world needs us. How's that? The world needs people with vision and drive. At any rate, what have we got to lose? Only life itself.

Bacon/Sausage

I want so much to believe these two heavily processed meats are not bad for us. I love them so much. It's been well-established that processed meat is bad. (Pardon the simplistic adjective "bad," but I see no solid reason to mince words when the evidence is conclusive.) However, a few stalwart and stubborn voices—including Davis and Teicholz—insist that a little bacon and sausage now and then won't kill us. Maybe not. Many others—including proponents of most diets that include or encourage eating meat—make no mention whatsoever of their potential carcinogenic effects. It's one of those areas where a spartan, rigid, unwavering exclusion may not be necessary. Or...you may be playing with fire.

Dairy

I'm just going to say this one more time. I probably don't even need to since this Appendix is named Bones of Contention, but I can't overstate and barely overcome the frustration I feel over reading such radically vehement opposing views about so many things. And dairy is one of the biggest. I need not repeat what I detailed in the text, but only recapitulate a few things. Eggs okay. Milk? Oh my gosh. Cottage cheese? Butter? Yogurt? Holy cow. Better not have any of them. Or...you better eat and drink lots of them. But better be sure they're all low or no fat if you do. Or, better be sure to avoid low-fat and eat full only whole, 100% high fat or nothing at all. Crazy confusion and all the authorities have convincing arguments. Each side is right and the other side is nuts. Full on comedy hour.

Diets

The choice is yours. With so many different ones—all claiming to be the best and right one—it comes down to two basic decisions: 1) to consume meat and dairy or not and, if so, how much; and 2) to go with a high or low carb approach.

Exercise

For most people, the objective with exercise is to lose weight and/or fat, gain muscle, and help your heart stay healthy with 20 minutes of cardio. The challenge is how best to lose weight and fat, and burn calories, while retaining and gaining muscle mass. If you don't need to lose weight, then it's another set of goals. The debates revolve around how much is too much and the merits of high-intensity vs. low-intensity.

Fat

The debate over high-fat vs. low-fat dairy and meat rages. As does just how harmful saturated fat actually is for us. No one questions the horrors of trans fat.

Grain

The case against grain is pretty convincing. Dr. Gundry, Dr. Davis, Dave Asprey...the list goes on. Grain contains lectins and gluten and glyphosate and several other really bad things for you. It's unnatural to eat, destroys your gut biome, makes you fat and hungry, and generally leads to a premature death. Bread and cereal are the two main forms that grain takes. White bread is the worst. Whole wheat has its proponents but could be just as bad as the white stuff since it has more grain than its heavily processed white cousins. Rice is nice according to billions of people, including lots of the "experts," yet it's also a grain and has many vocal prosecutors.

Meat

To eat or not to eat. Perhaps no other bone is more contended than this one.

Protein

Can we get enough protein just from our food? That depends on what food we eat and how much protein we decide we need. If not for the general state of radical disagreement over almost everything related to diet, exercise, and healthcare, it would be shocking how hard it is to get a good understanding about the pros and cons of this amount and source of protein vs. that amount and source. Personally, I don't think we do get enough protein from just our food—unless we eat lots of meat and dairy. So, a 40-50 gram protein shake or two each day may be a good idea. Or it might not.

Supplements

See the Appendix for my own curated short list of recommended supplements. Absolutely consult with your doctor and try the ones she and you feel are best for you. Do not accept my recommendations without thoroughly researching them yourself. Be sure to carefully read all the ingredients to be sure you're not taking too much of a particular vitamin because many supplements come with added B-12 or D-3, for example.

APPENDIX B

The Drill

By now, we should all know what we need to do. Let's call it "The Drill." If we follow this Drill religiously, we *will* live longer and better.

Although there are no 100% surefire "Preventions" or proven "Cures" for all that ails us, we can definitely make a lot of progress in the right direction toward living a longer, healthier life by doing the following to reduce inflammation and activate our longevity genes through hormesis and autophagy:

Avoid these:

- Excess sugar. After cigarettes, it's the #1 killer. Cancer cells love it. It's their fuel. That should tell you everything you need to know about it. And artificial sweeteners aren't much better.

- Processed food

- Lectins (See the Gut Biome in Chapter 2: Eating)

- Trans fat

- Vegetable oils

- Fried foods

- Proton Pump Inhibitors (PPIs): prevacid, omenprezole, and the like.

- Grains

- Antibiotics: they kill so many of your good bacteria, they're *"the equivalent of a bomb going off in your gut"* (Gundry, p. 30). Sometimes you need them, but definitely not for colds or the flu, for which they aren't effective anyway.

- Sitting, reacting, laziness, lethargy, too much TV and electronics, Social Media, negativity

Strive for caloric restriction and a proven diet

Eat less and follow a good diet plan, such as WW in conjunction with the Mediterranean diet of nutrient-dense foods that contain antioxidants.

Practice intermittent fasting.

It's absolutely essential. Recall Dr. Sinclair's #1 piece of advice to live longer and better: *"Eat less often."*

Eat more organic vegetables.

Since toxicity, oxidation, and inflammation can all contribute to DNA damage, eat more vegetables for their antioxidant and anti-inflammatory qualities. Be sure they are organic whenever possible.

Eat sirtuin-rich foods

Such as blackcurrants, kale, olives, olive oil, parsley, capers, onions, and fish (especially salmon and tuna) .

Eat foods rich in antioxidants

Such as vitamin C (red peppers, kale), anthocyanins (blueberries) and polyphenols (dark chocolate, cloves).

Drink green tea.

An excellent brand is Zabba's Organic Pu Erh Tea.

Olive Oil

Take 2 tbsp. of polyphenol-rich Olive Oil every day

Be Disciplined

Be Productive Every Day: know your Purpose, follow your MS, pursue your Goals, live by Principles.

Exercise every day

With at least 4 days a week devoted to high-intensity and cardiovascular exercise. Move. Stand up. Stretch. Walk. Ride a bike. Do yoga. Don't be sedentary!

Try cold therapy.

Take ice baths, cold showers, swim in cold lakes and oceans. *"Activate the mitochondria...by being a bit cold.... Take a brisk walk on a winter day in just a T-shirt... Exercise in the cold... Leave a window open overnight... Don't use a heavy blanket while you sleep"* (Sinclair, p. 110).

Stoke the Serotonin

Release this beast as often as you can. It's the key hormone that stabilizes our mood, feelings of well-being, and happiness. This hormone impacts our entire body. Exercise releases it and the amino acid tryptophan (See Amino Acids in Appendix D: Supplements) converts to serotonin in the brain. It's also released by getting up and getting going early in the morning.

Meditate and practice conscious breathing

Don't skip this part of the Drill. Mindfulness helps you do everything else in this Drill. It reduces stress and inflammation, two killers. Return to the breath. Note and observe your thoughts and emotions. Don't get caught up in them. Be the still, serene soul sitting on the riverbank watching the raging rapids surge continually by, carrying your thoughts and emotions downstream in the current without you going along with them.

Take supplements.

See Appendix D for suggestions.

<u>Sleep 8 hours every night.</u>

7-9 hours will work. Just get a really good sleep . Every. Single. Night.

<u>Follow this *PEERLESS* system.</u>

It's all laid out for you. Being productive, reading, and learning are also proven to increase your chances of a healthier, longer life. Stay on top of the latest information. Take charge of your life. You *can* live longer and better if you stick to it.

APPENDIX C

Biotracking Tools

If you're "all-in" and want to invest some money in learning more about your body and current state of health, quite a few companies can help you. Biotracking your biomarkers and hacking a better plan and results for yourself is a real eye-opener. I'm only going to list the companies and their products and services that I've used myself. So this is not an exhaustive list of what's available. I'm going to tell you about each one and let you know what I think of them.

Apple Watch

It took me a long time to decide to go back to wearing a watch. I was not sold on the idea or the value of this watch. But I broke down, got one, and like it. Can't say that I love it because it's a bit awkward to wear. However, it does mark and track my workouts and heartbeat and blood oxygen and a few other things. Its best feature, for me, is the sleep tracking. It tells me how well or poorly I slept. It's usually on par with how I feel that I slept, but sometimes it tells me I slept poorly when I feel like I slept well. So, that conflicting information and its extensive feedback gives you something to consider. Overall, as a biotracker, it does what it's supposed to do. I can live with the mild discomfort of wearing it in exchange for the valuable tracking. It's up to you to decide just how many markers you want to collect and track. By the way, get the cheapest one. I had the aluminum at first and then spent an extra $400 for the titanium and I can't see much difference at all, except that it's bulkier and heavier, which is not a good thing.

Autophagy

A physiological process that maintains homeostasis or normal functioning of the cells. You can hack it, if not track it, through the stress of intermittent fasting, exercise, and cold therapy. Drinking coffee also works. When your metabolism does not have the stored resources to satisfy the demands of fasting, exercise, exposure to cold, and coffee, autophagy will allow it to recycle damaged parts for energy and building materials. If it's good for your cells, it's good for you.

BioViva

For $467, they do a "TimeKeeper™ DNA Methylation" analysis. The only feedback you get is a few paragraphs telling you how old you are according to their "Longevity Clock" and their "Precision Chronological Clock." I'm 70 years old, but 63 by their LC and 58 by their PCC. That's nice. It's encouraging. But...where's the more extensive feedback? What does it mean? How have I scored this well? What can I expect? What can I continue to do or do better or more of? Tell me something more besides giving me 2 numbers for $467. I emailed them 3x expressing this concern, but to date they've haven't replied. I'd recommend spending your money elsewhere, such as with InsideTracker. https://biovault.bioviva-science.com

23&Me

An essential starting point is to have your DNA analyzed. They do so and provide you a full health breakdown for just $399. It's really priceless. Their reports are so extensive you'll be blown away at what you learn about your ancestry and lineage. Fascinating. https://www.23andme.com/

Dexafit

With 2 dozen locations in the US, I'd highly recommend you visit the one nearest you. For $299, you get 4 complete body scans—the initial one and

3 follow ups 2-3 months apart to measure your progress. The scans and reports measure your BMI and other markers, including visceral fat, the big one. Your visceral fat is the killer fat that collects around your internal organs. You want to reduce your VF as much as possible. Mine is in the high-risk range. Not good. I'm continuing the Drill, which is the best and only way to attack the problem. We'll see next month if I've made any progress. A solid investment. https://www.dexafit.com/

Everlywell

Good, inexpensive at-home testing of many markers, including metabolism, thyroid, and allergies, plus many more. https://www.everlywell.com/

Genopalate

For $69.95, they analyze what you should eat and what supplements you should take based on your existing DNA data (assuming you already have it from 23&Me or Ancestry). The reports and resources are interesting, but the drawback, to me, are the recommendations that I eat lots of carbs, including "starchy grains," that corn and canola oil are good for me, and that all legumes, including peanuts, are "great," among other standard, basic food groups notions. Don't think so. I'll pass. Thus, I believe that their feedback is dubious at best. https://genopalate.com

Elite HRV

As I already reviewed in Chapter 6 Exercise, HeartMath Solutions Coresense HRV measures that very important biomarker. I strongly recommend you look into it. https://elitehrv.com/

Inside Tracker

This company is the superstar of the bunch. By purchasing its $599 package, you get blood work on 24 essential biomarkers. Its feedback and reports are second to none, with extensive, full color breakdowns of your various levels, what it all means and what you can do to correct poor results. If you already have a DNA analysis—from 23&Me or Ancestry—the package also analyzes all of your bloodwork against your DNA and provides another comprehensive 40 page report. They also have a Facebook group and a wide variety of other services and support. One of the best $600 investments I've ever made. https://www.insidetracker.com

NAC

Use Neuro-Associative Conditioning (NAC) to train our brains to seek pleasure and avoid pain through simple reinforcement. You can *"Condition your nervous system to associate pleasure to those things you want to continuously move toward and pain to those things you need to avoid"* (Robbins, p. 112). Every time we recognize that what seems pleasurable is actually painful—eg. eating the wrong food, being lazy and skipping exercise to watch TV, indulging in too much alcohol or some stupid drug—we should mindfully pause, make a note of it, and engage in positive self-talk. Just tell ourselves how well we're doing. *That was good. I made the right decision. I did the right thing.* Meditate on it, on how you identified the pain disguised as pleasure.

RAS

Count on and activate your Reticular Activating System (RAS) by continually recalling and focusing hard on your goals and priorities. It bears repeating that your RAS will do the rest: *"Once you decide that something is a priority, you give it tremendous emotional intensity, and by continually focusing on it, any resource that supports its attainment will eventually become clear"* (Robbins, p. 287-288).

Scale

Get a $25-30 bathroom scale that measures BMI, Body Fat, Muscle Mass, Body Water, Visceral Fat and more. I have two different ones just because I was skeptical of their accuracy and wanted to check them against each other. They come up with almost identical numbers, so they seem accurate. Their numbers also match those from Dexafit. They're a great way to track these biomarkers right at home on an app.

Inevifit is my recommendation: https://www.inevifit.com/

TeloYears

They measure how old you are in telomere-years. The test isn't too expensive but the results take a while. I'm still waiting…. https://www.teloyears.com/home/

Time Management Matrix (TMT)

Study Covey's TMT to determine how you spend and prioritize your daily activites. Many of your Quadrant #2 activities are more important than you've previously thought, such as working on your self-improvement, learning, mindfulness, and meditation. Trying moving them to Quadrant #1—making them urgent.

	URGENT	NOT URGENT
IMPORTANT	Quadrant #1 **"NECESSITY"** ——— Your Key Action: **"MANAGE"** ——— **Common Activities** - Crises - Deadline-driven activities - Medical emergencies - Other "true" emergencies - Pressing problems. - Last minute preparations	Quadrant #2 **"QUALITY & PERSONAL LEADERSHIP"** ——— Your Key Action: **"FOCUS"** ——— **Common Activities** - Preparation and planning - Values clarification - Empowerment - Relationship-building - True recreation
NOT IMPORTANT	Quadrant #3 **"DECEPTION"** ——— Your Key Action: **"USE CAUTION or AVOID"** ——— **Common Activities** - Meeting other people's priorities and expectations - Frequent interruptions: - Most emails, some calls - Urgency masquerading as importance	Quadrant #4 **"WASTE"** ——— Your Key Action: **"AVOID"** ——— **Common Activities** - Escapist activities - Mindless tv-watching - Busywork - Junk mail - Some emails - Some calls

Adapted from Stephen Covey's "First Things First" - Covey Leadership Center, Inc. © 2003

APPENDIX D

Supplements

DISCLAIMER: I am not a doctor, so I cannot recommend what you should take. Check with your doctor before you take anything. Do not accept my recommendations without thoroughly researching them yourself. Be sure to carefully read all the ingredients to be sure you're not taking too much of a particular vitamin because many supplements come with added B-12 or D-3, for example.

That said, here's my own curated short list of recommended supplements. When applicable, I'll recommend an exact blend and "name brand" manufacturer. Again, these are just my own preferred products and you and your doctor must decide what's right for you.

Amino Acids

Take a good blend of the 8 essential ones. They produce protein, aid in muscle mass production, and speed recovery of your muscles after a workout. Be sure your blend includes tryptophan because it converts in your brain to serotonin—the absolutely essential hormone that facilitates cellular communication and aids in sleeping, digestion, mood, and happiness. I use Perfect Amino by Bodyhealth. 5000-10000 mg. per day.

Apple Cider Vinegar with Prebiotics

Its antioxidant effects are legendary: reducing cholesterol, lowering blood sugar levels, and improving symptoms of diabetes. It also enhances your energy, cleanses and detoxifies, and aids in weight loss by triggering ketosis, the process that occurs when your body burns fat for fuel. I use KETO + Apple Cider Vinegar by Purely Optimal. 1500 mg. daily.

Astragalus

An antioxidant herb used in traditional Chinese medicine for centuries, it boosts the immune system, reduces chronic inflammation, and helps the body contend with physical, mental, and emotional stress. Contained in TA-65 (see below)

BCAA

After a workout, take BCAA (Branched Chain Amino Acids) powder. It contains as its main ingredient L-Leucine: *"Of the 20 different amino acids, only leucine can activate a gene transcription factor, mammalian target rapamycin (mTOR), which increases protein synthesis in your muscles, and therefore helps build muscle and prevent the loss of muscle as you age"* (Asprey, *Game Changers*, p. 179). Available online or in health food stores.

Berberine

A newly discovered antioxidant—though used for thousands of years in Asian medicine –berberine is a natural alkaloid found in dozens of the world's most potent medicinal plants, including goldenseal and barberry. More than 4,000 studies have been published on berberine's remarkable health-boosting effects, such as reducing trigylcerides, improving metabolism and energy, lowering blood pressure, boosting cognitive function, aiding digestion, promoting weight loss, turbocharging the immune system, and inhibiting oxidative stress and inflammation of the liver, pancreas and kidneys. Wow. Many brands and formulas to choose from.

C

This mainstay vitamin is a strong antioxidant that can reduce the risk of heart disease, lower your blood pressure, and strengthen your immune system. I swear by its potent ability to help ward off the common cold. In my 20s and 30s, I had one cold after another. 7-10 a year. I was almost always sick. But in my late 30s, a friend told me to take 10000 mg. at the first sign of a cold coming on. So I tried it. I took 10000 mg and flooded my system with water. 5-6 hours later I took another 10000 mg and lots more water. The next day, I was fine. No cold. I had never before been able to stop a cold coming on. But that time, Vitamin C and water stopped it dead in its tracks. Since then, roughly 50% of the time it works: the cold symptoms are gone the next day and I feel perfectly well. A 50% success rate. It may not work for you, but it definitely works for me. The rest of the time, take 1000-2000 mg daily.

Collagen

Improves skin elasticity, increases bone density, reduces inflammation, thus lessening joint, back and knee pain, boosts gut health, and helps with weight loss and reducing body fat. Be sure the supplement includes Types I & III. 1750 mg daily.

CoQ10/Ubiquinol

In our bodies, CoQ10 converts to Ubiquinol which fights excess free radicals and helps protect our cells from damage. But because CoQ10 does not dissolve well, the body doesn't absorb as much of it as we need. Thus, a far superior CoQ10 supplement is one in which the CoQ10 has already been converted to Ubiquinol. A good brand is Qunol. 100 mg daily.

D3

D3 helps your body absorb calcium and phosphorus, important for building and keeping strong bones. It also helps support a healthy brain, heart, teeth, lungs, and immune system. 5000 IU daily.

DHEA

Inducing *"a range of youth promoting processes"* (*Transcend,* p. 77), it controls cortisol levels, slows the aging process, improves sports performance, enhances libido, promotes weight loss, bolsters the immune system, boosts testosterone levels, increases muscle mass and reduces fat mass. 50 mg daily.

Fisetin

An antioxidant, anti-inflammatory flavonoid polyphenol, it acts as a senolytic—meaning senescence destroying—removing senescent "zombie" cells, resulting in far better health and longevity. 100-500 mg daily.

Fish Oil (EPA/DHA)

It supports cardiovascular system health, by helping to maintain healthy triglyceride levels and normal blood pressure. It also reduces chronic inflammation, helps weight loss, and improves brain and liver function. 2000 mg daily.

Garlic

A powerful antioxidant, it reduces chronic inflammation, lowers blood pressure, improves cholesterol levels, and may even help prevent the common cold. 1000 mg daily.

Glucosamine Chondroitin with MSM

Supports healthy joints and reduces pain for those with osteoarthritis and other inflammatory joint problems. 1500 mg daily.

Glutamine

After a workout, take a Glutamine supplement powder. Exercising depletes your body's store of this amino acid that, like leucine, is essential in muscle recovery and growth. Available online or in health food stores.

Glutathione

Called "the Mother of Antioxidants," by protecting cells against free radicals, it reduces inflammation and fights oxidative stress, thereby slowing the aging process. Mitochondria *"depend heavily on glutathione for their well-being. In fact, scientists measure the levels of glutathione within mitochondria as an indicator of their vitality"* (Perlmutter, p. 120-121). 500 mg. daily.

Gut Health

1. Total Restore is Dr. Gundry's proprietary blend of all-natural ingredients that combats a leaky gut and promotes "a healthy gut lining." I'm a believer in Dr. Gundry, so I take it as directed.

2. Probiotics: "Friendly" or "good" bacteria, they balance out or even kill some "bad" bacteria, thus helping with digestion, constipation, IBS, cellular health, and general inflammation. I use Dr. Gundry's 24 Strain Probiotics.

3. Sodium Butyrate supports digestive health, helps control inflammation, promotes weight loss, and even aids in preventing disease. Many brands to choose from.

4. Lectin Guard. We discussed at length just how bad lectins are for your gut and general body health. A few supplements have proprietary blends of all-natural ingredients that promise to block lectins and improve digestion. I use Lectin Guard by KaraMD. 1800 mg daily.

K2

By aiding in the metabolism of calcium, it supports both bone and heart health. Dave Asprey even argues that it aids ALL other vitamins and minerals in doing their work (*Game Changers*, p. 193). 100 mg daily.

Magnesium

Important for many processes in the body, it regulates muscle and nerve function, blood sugar levels, and blood pressure, and helps make protein and improve bone health. 400 mg daily.

Metformin

A doctor's prescription needed, it's a Diabetes drug with great potential to impact many other conditions. Dr. Sinclair recommends it and is spearheading the Targeting Aging with Metformin (TAME) clinical trials to prove that it may influence metabolic and cellular processes that are associated with the development of age-related conditions. If your doctor will prescribe it, take it. 1000 mg daily.

MSM

Its anti-inflammatory properties decrease joint pain, aid in muscle recovery, alleviate arthritis and allergy symptoms, boost the immune system, improve your skin, fight lectins, and even help prevent cancer. 3000 mg daily.

Pterostilbene

A potent antioxidant that improves cellular, neurological, and cardiovascular health, regulates blood sugar and metabolism, aids in weight reduction, and lowers stress. 200 mg daily.

Resveratrol

An NAD+ booster to activate the Sirtuin pathway, Resveratrol is a polyphenol that may help prevent cancer and heart disease. Produced by grapes experiencing stress, it helps reduce hunger and, thus, restrict your caloric intake. *"When combined with intermittent fasting, it can greatly extend both average and maximum lifespan even beyond with fasting alone accomplishes"* (Sinclair, p. 133).

SAMe

Involved in the formation, activation, or breakdown of other chemicals in the body, including hormones, proteins, and certain drugs, SAMe helps with depression, osteoarthritis, anxiety, back pain, fibromyalgia, liver detoxification, and many other conditions. 400 mg daily.

Saw Palmetto

It helps increase testosterone levels, improves prostate health, reduces inflammation, prevents hair loss, and enhances urinary tract function. 2000 mg daily.

Selenium

It helps with regulating the metabolism, improving thyroid function, protecting the body from oxidative stress, boosting the immune system, slowing age-related mental decline, and even reducing the risk of heart disease. 200 mg daily.

TA-65

Its bioenhanced astragalus—steroidal molecules extracted from the root of the astragalus plant—is a clinically-proven telomerase activator. Developed and sold by T. A. Sciences, https://www.tasciences.com/, TA-65 isn't cheap, but its science is backed by more than 20,000 published articles. Dr. Fossel reports that in two studies conducted on people who have taken TA-65, *"there was evidence that telomere lengths were affected in most patients, and in both studies there was evidence of 'rejuvenation'"* (184). In one of our conversations, Dr. Fossel said he takes two 250mg. capsules every morning on an empty stomach. If that's what he does, that's what I'm doing. He's the man.

Tea, specifically Pu-erh tea

Made from the same plant as black and green tea, it is rich in polyphenols and other bioactive molecules that support immune health. It also helps with weight loss, stress, energy levels, and detoxification. I recommend Zabba's Organic. One 8oz glass per day.

Testosterone Booster

Low Testosterone levels causes belly fat gain, loss of strength, low libido, and muscle loss. A booster helps your body produce more natural Testosterone, leading to more lean muscle gains, faster fat loss, and a greater libido. Two independent websites rank TestoGen as the #1 supplement.

Timeline's Mitopure

A clinically proven nutrient that can "*revitalize mitochondria and power muscle cells*," it comes in either pill form or convenient, great-tasting packets you can add to a shake or smoothie. I'm sold on it. https://www.time-linenutrition.com/

TruNiagen

Backed by many clinical studies, its an NAD+ booster that activates the Sirtuin pathway, thereby helping with cellular energy and repair, cholesterol levels, and liver functioning. 600 mg daily.

Tumeric

A powerful antioxidant, it reduces chronic inflammation, and also shows evidence of helping to ease the symptoms of hay fever, depression, high cholesterol, itching, heartburn, and stress. 1000 mg daily.

Zinc

An essential mineral, it reduces chronic inflammation and is needed for DNA synthesis, immune function, metabolism and growth. 50-100 mg daily.

INDEX